Unveiling Lyme Disease

Is This What's Behind Your Chronic Illness?

By Lisa Dennys

IWI

Integrated Wellness
International Inc.

Cover Design: Amanda Downey
Editing: Kate Makled & Shannon Conway
Author's Photo Courtesy of Lorrie Williams

Integrated Wellness International Inc.
Sarnia, Ontario, Canada
www.unveilinglyme.com · info@unveilinglyme.com

Dedication

This book is dedicated to the countless people suffering with chronic illness due to undiagnosed Lyme Disease. May you never give up in your quest for satisfying answers and glorious recovery.

Advance Praise

Unveiling Lyme Disease is a well written and researched, plain talk patient guide to diagnosis, treatment, and day-to-day coping with the "great imitator", Lyme disease. Dennys, a former occupational therapist and Chinese medicine and acupuncture practitioner, provides a clear and compassionate roadmap for navigating tick-borne diseases especially for Canadian patients. Readers will be especially moved by her own harrowing 30-year struggle to finding answers for her multiple symptoms and her lessons will be helpful for the hundreds of thousands of others struggling with tick-borne and other chronic disease. I highly recommend this book.

— Dr. Richard I. Horowitz MD, medical director, Hudson Valley Healing Arts Center, author of *Why Can't I Get Better? Solving the Mystery of Lyme and Chronic Disease,* and *How Can I Get Better? An Action Plan for Treating Resistant Lyme & Chronic Disease.* Founding Member of ILADS

Lisa Dennys is about to take you on a journey that will change your life. Her genuineness asks us each to consider what lengths we are really willing to go, to become the

"General Contractor" of our own health. She educates us about the realities and shortcomings of our health care systems and this mysterious disease with practicality and common sense. Rather than complaining or giving up, she provides top-notch skills and practical solutions for advocating for yourself, all the while managing day-to-day exhaustion. This book need be applied to all chronic health issues. You will gain an ally and real skills to find the right resources for your own complex health situation. What I appreciated the most is Lisa sharing the graphic and very real heroics of living with, let alone championing any chronic condition. This passionate voice sharing what people truly experience has been long overdue. This book is humbling and inspiring and should be mandatory reading for every human being.

— Lori Wilson, author of *Demystifying…Medical Intuition*, Founder of *Inner Access 101*

Unveiling Lyme Disease by Lisa Dennys is a succinct, user-friendly guide that will fast track your search for finding the answers and help that you need to get you on the road to healing. She not only helps you free up the shame associated with chronic illness by validating your struggle, but also works to empower you with step by step directions for cutting through the confusion of diagnosis, and the development of your healthcare plan. If you are suffering from symptoms that will not resolve and are beginning to suspect Lyme disease, I recommend this book as your first step to empowerment and healing.

— Nancy Raymond, MSMS, MS, RDN, FAARFM, Optimal Health Solutions, *LLC*, Advanced Fellow in Anti-aging, Regenerative and Functional Medicine, A4M, Integrative and Functional Medicine RDN

In *Unveiling Lyme Disease*, Lisa empowers the individual and their families by explaining the scope of Lyme disease and co-infections (it's everywhere!), exposing many of the misdiagnoses resulting from Lyme disease (fibromyalgia, chronic fatigue syndrome, Parkinson's disease, ALS, unexplained neurological and neuropsychiatric symptomatology, and many other syndromes); offering tips on how to navigate the medical system, and explaining the benefits of self–advocating.

Lisa also advises the reader on various aspects of self-care and methods to recover from debilitating chronic illnesses through practical examples from her own experiences on the road to healing from Lyme disease.

This work is accurate and refreshing as it flies in the face of traditional medical thinking and practice by showing the suffering individual and their families that there is a root cause to their chronic illness and, most of all, a path to true healing.

I found *Unveiling Lyme Disease: Is This What's Behind Your Chronic Illness?* accurate, engaging, full of practical and immediately useful information and, most of all, a beacon of hope for all who suffer but know not why.

—Dr. Jess P. Armine, The Center for Bio-Individualized Medicine

Undiagnosed Lyme disease is one of the most devastating experiences for anyone with a health issue, in large part because of how difficult it is to uncover this elusive disease. Lisa's book is desperately needed for those on this journey.

In a very personal journey towards greater medical self-advocacy, Lisa provides practical coping skills needed for navigating a new diagnosis while gently caring for mind, body and spirit. *Unveiling Lyme Disease* is an essential guide for those who persevere to find a new path to recovery.

A missed diagnosis of Lyme creates long term frustrating and debilitating consequences in the lives of so many who are suffering with a chronic illness which is actually treatable. In a sensitive, enlightening and empowering way, Lisa gives hope for those who persevere in finding the expert answers and supportive help they need to enter a new path of self-advocacy, leading to recovery of mind, body and spirit.

— Joyce O'Brien, Speaker, Vitality Specialist and Author of #1 Bestseller *Choose to Live: Our Journey from Late Stage Cancers to Vibrant Health*

I am not only a practitioner, but like many others have travelled a long and winding road in my own health journey, going to countless specialists, wondering if I would ever get well. *Unveiling Lyme Disease* provides valuable information to help prevent and avoid pitfalls that people with chronic illness commonly experience, even while doing their best to stay positive. This book is a must to read if you are not getting answers or feel you have been bounced from specialist to specialist. I wish this book had been around years ago, to help me find my way through the darkness and into the light.

— Shawn Bean, Specialist in Clinical Nutrition, Matrix Health and Wellness LLC, The Center for Bio-Individualized Medicine

Table of Contents

Introduction

"In the fullness of time, the mainstream handling of chronic Lyme disease will be viewed as one of the most shameful episodes in the history of medicine because elements of academic medicine, elements of government and virtually the entire insurance industry have colluded to deny a disease. This has resulted in needless suffering of many individuals who deteriorate and sometimes die for lack of timely application of treatment or denial of treatment beyond some arbitrary duration."[1]
— Kenneth B. Liegner, M.D.

As I imagine the reason you've picked up this book, I suspect you have spent months or even years of your life feeling lousy, losing pieces of yourself, your health, your work, and your relationships to an illness that is elusive, mysterious and disruptive.

I can't stand to watch you blame yourself for being wrong, weak or flawed for not being able to overcome a condition you don't even yet know that you may have.

I'm writing this book to introduce you to the possibility that the struggles that you have had with your health that you have been told are due to chronic fatigue syndrome or fibromyalgia, maybe even MS or ALS, may actually be undiagnosed chronic Lyme disease. Or the vague collection of symptoms that is yet to be diagnosed as anything other than aches, pains and worries–you feel awful and cannot function, yet the doctors can find nothing wrong. That, too, may be undiagnosed chronic Lyme disease.

Yes, Lyme disease.

There are lots of reasons why this can happen to people like you and why you don't know yet that it's what you really are struggling with.

I know you have your suspicions that all is not what it appears to be in your health picture.

I know that Lyme disease has been in the news a lot lately and that when you come across articles with those huge symptom lists, you see yourself in those lists and start to wonder: "Could that be me, too?" Maybe you have suspected it, but then dismissed the idea.

I know you are fed up with the state of your health, and you are someone who wants to look deeper for answers. You don't give up easily. You're made of tough stuff. That's how you've made it this far in your life.

In this book, I'm going to show you where you need to place your efforts so you can find out — once and for all — what is going on. I'm going to let you know why it's still possible — and not unusual — for you to have undiagnosed Lyme disease, despite having seen countless experienced and competent medical specialists already.

Are you angry and incredulous at the possibility that what I'm saying is true? That it really is possible for you to have Lyme disease, even if you have had the standard Lyme testing and been told, "You're fine"?

I don't blame you. I was angry, too, when decades of

misdiagnosis happened to me, and when chronic Lyme disease turned out to be my reality. At the same time, what I have learned about coping with chronic illness and the capacity I have regained once started on effective treatment, has inspired me to reach as many people as possible with hope, coping strategies, and a realistic plan to get the answers you need to be well.

The Lyme Mystery

Lyme disease, a bacterial infection caused by the spirochete Borrelia burgdorferi, is transmitted primarily by the bite of a tick, which often carries other nasty co-infection — creating bacteria such as Bartonella, Babesia, Erlichia, Anaplasma, Rocky Mountain Spotted Fever, Mycoplasma, and is associated with viruses such as Epstein Barr, Cytomegalovirus, HHV-6 and others. Evidence suggests there may be other forms of transmission as well, such as sexual transmission.

But how can a known bacterial illness, commonly transmitted by the bite of a tiny tick, be a problem to detect, diagnose and treat? And in this time of modern medical miracles, how can it be such a growing concern that it is emerging as a significant public health epidemic, yet still be so vastly undetected that it can go on to become a serious, chronic and complex condition?

There are many reasons for this, which I'm going to discuss much more in this book.

The Scope of Lyme Disease: The Great Imitator

Lyme disease is rapidly becoming a "rampant epidemic in the 21st century".[2] According to the USA-based Centers for Disease Control (CDC) the incidence of Lyme disease in the USA has been estimated by to be as high as 376,000 new people per year.[3]

These alarming numbers rival those of HIV (50,000 new cases per year in the USA in 2014)[4] breast cancer[5] (224,147 new cases in USA in 2012) and colorectal cancer (134,784 cases in USA in 2012).[6] There are about 200 new cases of MS diagnosed in the USA each week and about 400,000 people are living with MS in the USA. Researchers are studying the potential connection between MS and infections.[7]

Due to its long and varied list of symptoms that may wax and wane, Lyme disease, called "the great imitator", can masquerade as many other common diseases and conditions.[8]

Due to the wide-ranging, multi-system and often inconsistent symptoms, physicians who are not familiar with the way that chronic Lyme disease presents will frequently misdiagnose Lyme by attributing the symptoms to another condition. Serious diseases such as MS, ALS, Parkinson's disease, various psychiatric illnesses, Alzheimer's disease and many others have been linked to Lyme disease.[9]

Chronic Fatigue Syndrome (CFS) or Fibromyalgia, whose diagnostic numbers are also growing, may also turn out to be examples of conditions caused by or linked to missed cases of Lyme disease.[10] Estimates of the number of people with CFS in the USA vary from 7 to 3,000 per 100,000 adults.[11] The incidence of Fibromyalgia is estimated to be one in 50 people in the USA.[12] There has been much research over the years looking for the possible microbes that may be at the root of these chronic and often debilitating conditions. More closely investigated cases of these mysterious syndromes have sometimes been attributed to Lyme disease in recent years.[13]

The co-existence of debilitating active viruses such as Epstein Barr virus (EBV), Cytomegalovirus (CMV), and human herpes virus 6 (HHV-6) as well as the accumulation of laboratory-verified environmentally-based toxins such as molds and heavy metals may also further complicate Lyme disease, resulting in (or due to) significant strain on the affected person's immune system.[14] It is hard to tell for certain whether there is cause or effect here, however each of these factors contributes to a health picture that is complicated and challenging for sure. A concerning number of people with autoimmune diseases such as Rheumatoid Arthritis, Crohn's Disease and Lupus have also been found to have Lyme disease.[15]

How many people are actually suffering with Lyme disease, a curable, bacteria-based illness, and how many go on to have serious or fatal complications because this illness was never diagnosed properly?

About 50% of people never develop the classic 'bulls-eye' rash after a painless tick bite.[16] So they (and their doctors, if consulted) never realize that the onset of typical Lyme symptoms such as flu-like complaints, fever, joint pain and swelling, headache, chills, nausea, dizziness, fatigue, sore throat, and swollen glands have had anything to do with a tick bite. Symptoms may present acutely and then disappear, only to return periodically weeks or even months later.[17]

Moreover, it is also theorized that Lyme is not only transmitted via tick bites after all, even though awareness of Lyme has primarily focused on awareness of tick bite prevention. So many people with Lyme never believed they were at risk because of that link.

Dr. Richard I. Horowitz, a renowned physician specializing in diagnosing and treating Lyme disease and its co-infections, and New York Times bestselling author of two books, *Why Can't I Get Better? Solving the Mystery of Lyme & Chronic Disease* and *How Can I Get Better? An Action Plan for Treating Resistant Lyme & Chronic Disease*, has developed a comprehensive patient assessment questionnaire. It includes 43 symptoms, risk assessment and a scoring system to help with Lyme disease screening. It is available on my webpage in your complimentary Quick Start Guide to Unveiling Lyme Disease here. Dr. Horowitz uses the term multiple systemic infectious disease syndrome (MSIDS) to describe the complex constellation of co-existing issues that Lyme patients and their physicians have to deal with.[18]

Another checklist that can be utilized to assess for Lyme symptoms, developed by Dr. Joseph J. Burrascano Jr., is available from the Canadian Lyme Disease Foundation website.

What about chronic Lyme disease?

The development of chronic Lyme disease, as a result of an undiagnosed or untreated case of acute Lyme, can create many years or even decades of waxing and waning (or more constant) multi-symptom illness. The consequences can be extreme, sometimes resulting in severe or even fatal neurological[19] or cardiac symptoms.[20]

Although there are many disturbing problems that arise from the challenges in accurately diagnosing acute Lyme disease, there are also big issues with identifying and treating chronic Lyme disease as well. There are controversial medical and political and issues around Lyme lab testing and diagnosis, as well as conflicting and wide-ranging ideas about treatment approaches. There is even controversy about whether chronic Lyme is a 'real' disease or not,[21] much to the frustration of those of us with chronic Lyme and the skilled doctors who are treating us. The International Lyme and Associated Diseases Society (ILADS) gives a list of 10 tips to prevent chronic Lyme disease.

The chronic illness problem: How does this systems-wide issue affect Lyme detection and treatment?

People with chronic illness make up a large percentage of those seeking diagnostic and treatment help in our already strained health care systems. Those seeking treatment for chronic illness account for 86% of the total USA health care costs[22] and 67% of total Canadian health care costs.[23] Three out of five Canadians over the age of 20 have some form of chronic disease.[24]

But this population gets woefully underserved, for many reasons that range from emphasis on the Western medical model, to complex funding issues, to attitudes of health care practitioners or the patients themselves.

The health care systems of first world countries have many strengths, but dealing with the complexities of chronic illness is not one of them. Most of our health care expertise is geared towards the diagnosis and treatment of emergency and acute conditions, for which drugs and surgery are the main forms of treatment. People with chronic illnesses often find themselves falling between the cracks of the system, because there is pressure to make quick decisions and alleviate symptoms. There are not enough resources allocated to truly determine the multi-faceted and complex root causes of any chronic condition.

I believe that effective treatment for chronic illness requires a varied team of health professionals and individualized attention, not recipes or cookie-cutter approaches administered in bite-sized office visits. Financial and time constrictions, limitations in medical training, and narrow views of what truly contributes to health and illness are just some of the many factors that leave chronic illness patients underserved, unheard and under-functioning.

So what does this all this have to do with you, and with the possibility that you may have Lyme disease? Problems within our medical systems that limit the ability to effectively deal with chronic illness as a whole, severely impact the access you may have to medical expertise in the diagnosis and treatment of chronic Lyme disease.

The problems with Lyme detection

The serious medical and political controversy about Lyme disease testing and treatment is having a devastating effect on those affected by this debilitating condition.

Some medical organizations, such as the US-based IDSA (Infectious Diseases Society of America) deny the existence of chronic Lyme disease, calling lingering symptoms "Post-Treatment Lyme Disease Syndrome", even in the absence of a history of acute diagnosis or treatment.[25]

Others, such as US-based ILADS (International Lyme and Associated Diseases), are working towards changing existing diagnosis and treatment guidelines to adequately address those with chronic Lyme, which they believe is a true concern and a serious, growing problem.[26]

The US-based CDC (Centers for Disease Control) has set strict guidelines for the diagnosis and treatment of Lyme for the USA (and upon which Canadian provincial health care standards are also based). Many physicians and patients remain frustrated by these guidelines, which are laced with very concerning issues.[27] These guidelines include inadequate standards for testing, (which often fails to accurately pick up the presence of existing acute or chronic Lyme disease), and limits to the length of time that physicians can prescribe antibiotic treatment.[28]

So-called Lyme literate physicians (LLMD's) object to the IDSA guidelines for very serious reasons, which they have encountered in medical practice. Treating acute Lyme for too short a time frame can result in its development into chronic Lyme disease.[29] There have been physicians who have been subject to disciplinary action or even forced to stop practicing medicine due to legal proceedings against them for treating chronic Lyme patients using long-term antibiotics. This is despite the long–term use of antibiotics (for months or years) being a common practice among Lyme specialists — and its frequently positive results in successfully returning better functional ability and quality of life to those afflicted with chronic Lyme.[30]

Another bigger 'systems' issue that explains why Lyme goes so often misdiagnosed, is simply the way our health care system is organized. We do not have access to many Lyme-informed "generalist specialists", an apt term coined by Dr. Jess Armine of the Center for Bio-Individualized Medicine. This is a word for skilled, Lyme literate professionals who are astute chronic illness problem solvers, and therefore able to assess complex cases in a very integrated and holistic way.[31]

Lyme requires a clinical diagnosis: a careful evaluation of a patient's history, physical examination, and very extensive lab work-ups with interpretation by a Lyme specialist. It requires experience to discern subtleties that an untrained mind misses. It is not a cut and dried, one-test diagnostic process.[32]

Our mainstream medical system is based on various specialties, each of which categorize, identify and treat the many malfunctions that can occur within that area of the body's anatomy and physiology. The body is assessed from the standpoint of these separate areas of function, like the brain and nervous system, the immune system, the heart, the hormonal system, and the reproductive system. Problems tend to be categorized as either physically-based illness to be addressed by specialists in the above disciplines, or as mentally based, and referred to psychiatrists.

Someone with as-yet-undiagnosed Lyme may typically be sent to one or many medical specialties for evaluation, depending upon which symptoms are primary, or most prominently featured. In order to give you access to the specialist, your family physician interprets what further specialty help may or may not be required, based upon his or her extensive (but potentially incomplete, when it comes to Lyme) training and experience. Referrals may be made to a wide range of distinct specialties, which means you may see one or more of the following: neurologist, rheumatologist, endocrinologist, gynecologist, psychiatrist, or cardiologist.

These specialties are highly trained to identify diseases and pathologies that fall clearly within their own fields. The broad list of Lyme disease symptoms, which is one that suggests trouble for multiple fields of expertise, simply does not fit into our existing model of mainstream medicine.

The result of *not* getting a Lyme diagnosis, when you do have Lyme disease? Here's what may happen to you, as has happened to others:

- Years of ongoing, needless illness and suffering.

- Lack of meaningful diagnosis to explain your symptom severity.

- Drug treatment with adverse side effects, treating a condition that is ultimately a wrong diagnosis, and not fixing the root problem that no one yet realizes you have.

- Worsening of your condition, sometimes with fatal consequences (such as heart failure, because the real cause, the underlying Lyme disease that has been progressively destroying your heart tissue, was never identified).

- Receiving a misdiagnosis of a condition that is seen as invariably progressive and incurable like MS, Alzheimer's or ALS, when the truth is a treatable case of infection with Lyme bacteria.

- An unknown fatality attributed to an unknown cause.[33]

- Being accused, by Lyme-unaware physicians, of malingering, the suggestion that it really is all in your head, or being told that you just have to live with it the best you can, because there is nothing more that can be done to explain let alone treat it.

- Years of blaming yourself, concluding that you must be making it all up: the self-image, social, occupational and relationship consequences of unexplained ill health.

As I have had the opportunity to learn and now teach, navigating successfully through this dilemma to get a reliable diagnosis of Lyme disease in the first place, and then starting into the successful process of recovery does not just 'happen'. *It requires specific skill development, and bold action.* But there is hope in the pure fact that it involves *learned skills*, not some magical innate ability or luck.

The skills you will need to build are in three key areas: navigating the medical system, maximizing your day-to-day functioning, and acknowledging the role your mind and spirit will play in helping you on your road to recovery. These skills will help you find your way out of this mess and back into the kind of great life you may have given up on ever having again.

Living with undiagnosed Lyme disease has a major impact on your quality of life. It impacts the way you feel about yourself, and in turn that dictates the way you may push yourself to exhaustion to keep going, perhaps because you have been told there's "nothing wrong", despite the symptoms that are severely limiting you. It impacts your work, your quality of life and all of your relationships.

This impact physically, emotionally and financially for those with undiagnosed Lyme and their families, is brutal — and unnecessary. It happened to me, and it has impacted my husband, and every aspect of our life together for the past 30 years. I don't want it to happen to you. I want to show you how you can save a lot of time, money, suffering and anguish. I want to show you that you can take the steps you will need to take, to find the root of your undiagnosed illness and to ultimately return to the kind of health and life you've been missing.

That is why I am writing this book, and why I want to reach as many of you as I possibly can.

Chapter 1: Getting a Diagnosis
Finding Specialized Lyme Help

So now that I've introduced you to some of the complex issues involved in getting a Lyme diagnosis, you're likely wondering, "Now what? Where do I start?"

Before we start talking more specifically about Lyme disease symptoms and proceeding to information about testing and diagnosis, we need to look at a more basic issue. It can be a problem simply to get access to proper medical evaluation, so that you can find out, once and for all, if you actually do have Lyme disease or not.

The Lyme disease medical blind spot

Lyme disease is a new kid on the block, medically speaking. That's hard to believe when it seems to be plastered all over the news these days, right?

What do I mean by *new*?

In medicine, diseases, conditions, and phenomena are considered new if they were discovered within the last several decades. It takes a long time for patient care to catch up with medical research findings, even where investment and activity toward research is significant on a certain topic. A 2003 report stated that the delay between medical research discovery and clinical application of that discovery averaged 17 years.[34]

The training that typically takes place in medical schools is based on information from current clinical practice. But the amount of basic scientific research, as well as clinical medical research going on at any given time is staggering. There are new discoveries in Western medicine constantly, many of which show huge promise in direct patient application.

Where it gets backlogged is that the clinical research (where basic research is put into real life testing, or patient application) still has to be done. And the continual medical training for doctors in order to enable them to use those clinical research applications just can't keep up.

Physicians are bound by the standards of practice that have been set up by governing bodies based on *traditions* of education and practice. Get where I'm going here? This is all a very slow process — from discovering something significant, doing basic and clinical research, and finally putting something into clinical practice to hopefully help the patient. On a macro level, medicine is innovative. Today's patients, however, may still be years away from reaping the benefits of today's investigations. More on that in Chapter Three.

Some facts about Lyme Disease

The history of Lyme disease began in 1975 when a group of people in Lyme, Connecticut became ill with unique arthritic symptoms. By 1977, the transmission of this illness was linked to the black-legged tick. The Lyme-causing spiral-shaped bacteria, known as a spirochete, was identified and named *Borrelia burgdorferi* in 1982.[35]

That makes Lyme disease a fairly recent discovery in the medical world, even though as far back as 1918 a spirochete was identified in the brains of multiple sclerosis (MS) patients who had died.[36] Syphilis, also called "the great imitator" in the 19th century, is another example of a spirochete induced disease.[37]

Lyme disease is a vector-borne disease: it is transmitted primarily by the bite of a tick, or at least one which has become infected with the bacteria, normally by ingesting the blood of infected mammals such as deer or rodents. Various types of ticks, mosquitoes, spiders, fleas, chiggers, flies and mites can all carry Lyme disease-causing bacteria.[38] The bacteria in turn, in their new host, enter various organs and tissues throughout the body, including joints, brain, heart, and digestive system.[39]

Evidence suggests there may be other forms of Lyme transmission as well, such as sexual transmission.[40]

Lyme Symptoms

Lyme disease in its acute form can be notoriously difficult to detect. Symptoms of acute Lyme disease, following a bite from an infected tick, can occur anywhere from 24 hours to several weeks following the bite itself. Acute symptoms may range from very subtle to much more obvious at first. More severe symptoms such as intense headaches, joint pain and swelling, and heart and central nervous system problems can occur months or years later.[41]

Initial symptoms, such as fatigue, fever, headache, stiff

neck and joint and muscle pain may be so generalized in some cases that many people think they just have the flu, and Lyme is never even considered. It does not occur to them to seek medical help. Symptoms may even disappear completely for a time, leading the person to believe that they are fine, and support the hypothesis that they have recovered from the flu. That is another reason why, even in its acute form, Lyme is called "the great imitator."

Other people may have lingering symptoms, such as joint pain and swelling or arthritis, intermittent fever, fatigue, mood changes, headaches, heart or nervous system issues — and then they seek medical attention for all these things that never resolve. Commonly, they are told any number of reasons (or not) for this by their physician, who also has no clue it's Lyme, because Lyme is not even on the family doctor's radar.

Another complication with Lyme is that the infected tick may transmit other nasty diseases along with it. Each of these diseases comes with its own set of diverse symptoms, many of which also can be confused with other illnesses such as flu or various acute or chronic inflammatory conditions. A complete listing of these significant co-infections and their symptoms can be found at the *Canadian Lyme Disease Foundation* website: http://canlyme.com/just-diagnosed/co-infections/specific-co-infections/.

Although up to 30–50% of people who receive a tick bite may identify the characteristic bulls-eye rash, a larger percentage never notices a thing, and the bite itself is usually painless. You may never find a tick on you to require removal, nor any other sign that clues you in to the fact that there was ever any external invader. By the way, if you do find yourself with a tick attached to you, here are instructions for properly removing the tick and what to do next: http://canlyme.com/lyme-prevention/tick-removal/.

Your own Blind Spot, which can delay your Lyme diagnosis

Another challenge that can delay getting a Lyme diagnosis may be coming from your own mind. Yes, you read this right! *Your own mind can be in the way of finding out that you really may have Lyme.* How is this possible?

You may have grown so accustomed to the diagnosis that you were given (and may have even fought hard to have your symptoms believed enough by your doctors to finally get that diagnosis, *any* diagnosis), that it hasn't occurred to you to consider that it may be wrong.

You may have been struggling for years just trying to adapt to the daily challenges of living with something that you have been told is an incurable condition — like chronic fatigue syndrome or fibromyalgia or MS — and that has taken up all of your energy. As you kept trying to adapt yourself and your life to your limitations, the only thing that you may have ever considered to be wrong, faulty or not-good-enough has been you, rather than your diagnosis!

This was something that happened to me as well.

Before I got my chronic Lyme disease diagnosis in the spring of 2015, I spent years going to various health professionals. I was given a couple of labels for what was supposedly wrong with me. The prevalent label of chronic fatigue syndrome was the one that I had most internalized as being my primary condition. It was a vaguely known entity at best, and was an invisible ailment that had no obvious outside signs. No one looked further for a root cause of this, like an infection. It was just a syndrome, and that was it. There was no wondering *why* this was occurring. There was no sign of curiosity to try to do more than alleviate the disparate symptoms.

I looked fine to the outside world. I worked, attended a few social events, went home and collapsed. How my life looked on the outside was not how it really was on the inside.

I kept pretending to myself and to others that I must not really be sick, it must have just been that I was defective somehow, for not being able to cope with life like others appeared to be able to sustain. I would go through periods of time during which I *seemed* to be relatively OK, and could function relatively normally, as long as I kept pushing myself.

I convinced myself that it was normal to be too tired to do much of anything other than struggle through some basic household chores in the evenings and on the weekends, and withdraw from the world because it was too much effort to socialize. Inside, I was feeling ashamed and thought that I just wasn't trying hard enough to overcome what must be normal pain, exhaustion, insomnia, anxiety and many other symptoms. So I kept going, until I had yet another crash and was forced to stop working, again. This pattern would repeat itself for over 30 years.

It's not that I was not open to another diagnosis, because

I kept actively looking for answers. But that shameful view of myself that had gradually crept in without adequate answers was actually an impediment by this point. It made me think my condition was mostly my fault, a set of character flaws or constitutional inadequacy, not allowing room to insist that it could be anything like a *real, serious disease.*

Shame and doubt inhibited me from even learning more about Lyme online and considering it as a strong possibility for myself. I lost a lot of years of my life by not being aware of chronic Lyme disease and its far-reaching effects. It was never really on my radar.

Can't my family doctor take care of testing for Lyme to diagnose me?

So if you think you may have Lyme disease, isn't this just a simple matter of going to the doctor, getting tested and getting treated?

No, it's not.

And that is the crux of the challenge with Lyme disease. We need to backtrack a bit and differentiate between acute Lyme disease and chronic Lyme disease.

First, let's look at acute Lyme. If you're feeling sick and you see yourself in some of the symptom lists you've looked at, how do you know if you may have Lyme, and who do you seek out for help and when?

Here's a best case, but unfortunately rare, scenario. Let's say you've been out for a walk in the woods, you've come home and identified a tick that's partly embedded under your skin. You remove the offender, and you rapidly develop a bulls-eye rash and classic flu-like symptoms. You know this could be Lyme because you have read about it somewhere, or you know someone who has been worried they had it in the past. You get in to see your doctor right away, your doctor knows what to look for, and makes a clinical diagnosis of acute Lyme disease (i.e. no lab testing, just knowing from your signs, symptoms and history). Because this is a best-case scenario, she/he takes a professional risk and surpasses the current medical guidelines for how long to treat you with antibiotics, and gives you the correct antibiotic for a course lasting four or even six weeks. Then you get better, and you conclude that you have eradicated your Lyme disease.

Or, you may have unknowingly been dealing with acute Lyme disease at one point in time. But you thought it was the flu. You don't remember *ever* having a tick bite. The original symptoms seemed to go away, but then came back, as more symptoms seemed to layer on, making it unclear whether this was still the same problem, or a set of new ones. No one is at fault. You didn't know it could be Lyme. Your doctor didn't know, either. It was an innocent omission.

Chances are, you're reading this book because you're feeling awful and still looking for answers, so you've already missed the best case boat. The time period for identifying and treating acute Lyme disease has passed. Now, you may be into chronic Lyme disease territory.

If Lyme is the problem, that is why you may have lingering, worsening symptoms, or why the treatment for some other condition you've been told you have is still not working. That is why you may have been told to do one thing by one doctor and a different thing by another doctor.

This all may come as a bit of shock. Why am I talking this way? The usual process we've all been taught is supposed to go more like this:

1. You notice that your lingering health concern is not getting better.

2. You possibly have some ideas (or not) about what may be wrong, and what your diagnosis might be.

3. You go to your family physician, and you believe he or she will either know what is wrong and treat it him — or herself, or will send you to a specialist. This may or may not require some tests, and tests are always accurate, aren't they?

4. The specialist gets the test results, knows exactly what is wrong, and promptly diagnoses and treats you.

5. You follow the doctor's treatment recommendations, and then you recover.

End of story, right?

Since you're already dealing with chronic health problems, it's likely you've already found out in your medical travels that it's not that simple, for either the patient or the doctor. Having lived with chronic illness for a substantial period of time, you've already found out that this old paradigm hasn't worked for you so far. But you keep hoping that if you just hit the right, yet-unknown medical specialist, it will all get figured out, won't it? And perhaps you have an idea of who that ideal specialist might be, or if you are like a lot of us you might be stabbing in the dark or thinking it is a matter of luck or persistence.

If you do have Lyme, it *will* get figured out if you go to a Lyme specialist. But how do you access one of those professionals?

Can't my family doctor just do my testing and then refer me on to a Lyme specialist?

I wish it was that simple. So why *doesn't* your family doctor know that it may be chronic Lyme disease you're dealing with, do the testing herself/himself to confirm it, and then send you to a Lyme specialist for treatment? We're back to that Lyme disease blind spot in medical education I talked about earlier. Your family doctor may not really know to even consider Lyme disease. And due to your own blind spots, you may never have considered it, either.

The particular challenge with Lyme disease is that you can't count on the medical world, at least at your point of entry into the system, to know more about it than you do. This is where the responsibility lies on you to be your own health care advocate.

Lyme is not like many other conditions that are better known and more easily diagnosed, where you can count on your doctor having it incorporated into their everyday diagnostic thinking by default, in order to know to check for it.

In a perfect world, Lyme disease in its acute and chronic forms would be well known to all family doctors, and they would have Lyme specialists they would refer to. These Lyme specialists would commonly assess patients, referred by those family doctors, whom they have competently screened and suspect may have Lyme. But your family doctor may not even know that a Lyme specialist exists, or when to consult one.

In Canada, I don't know of any Lyme specialist medical doctors who are covered under provincial health insurance, and therefore a part of a referral network in mainstream medicine.

They just don't exist.

So if my family doctor can't send me to a Lyme specialist, what do I do now?

OK, it's now getting complicated. You're still sick, you wonder if you may have chronic Lyme, and you've passed the timeframe in which you could readily treat acute Lyme, even if you thought you may have had it, or if your family doctor even knew what to do with it.

You are likely going to have a lot of questions, and be feeling a lot of different emotions in response to this information so far. It's not easy to digest it all. The answer about what to do next and why is complicated too, so please bear with me on this. Instead of first just going to a doctor to give you answers, you need to learn more about the questions to ask, so that you know who to access and why.

You need to know more about what you may be dealing with: chronic Lyme disease.

Once you understand some key things about chronic Lyme disease, you'll be able to put some of these pieces together and feel more confident in your ability to get proper medical help. Accessing the right resources at the right time is critical, because as you've learned so far, this is not a simple process with Lyme.

The under-diagnosis of acute Lyme disease is one of the reasons chronic Lyme exists. The issue goes beyond the fact that family physicians are not trained to be on alert to identify acute or especially chronic Lyme disease. Insufficient length of treatment of acute Lyme, even if given a course of antibiotics, may result in a recurrence of Lyme infection due to incomplete eradication. This is known as Post-Treatment Lyme Disease, also embroiled in medical controversy as to what it is, why it occurs and how to treat it.

Some patients with chronic Lyme symptoms may never have antibodies show up on standard lab testing, despite lingering and debilitating illness. This makes detection of Lyme by commonly-used blood testing methods very difficult, resulting in the identification of Lyme disease often being completely missed.[42]

In the case of Lyme and co-infections, an additional significant challenge is that the bacteria are very ingenious and can mutate and hide out in various ways, often evading treatment attempts with either pharmaceutical antibiotics or naturally-sourced antimicrobials.

Another issue related to the emergence of Lyme, especially with no apparent connection to a tick bite, has to do with immune system stressors that may trigger the active expression of Lyme. The bacteria could have been lying dormant for years, where it has been kept at bay by your own immune system.

Due to various inter-related stressors, ranging from environmental (heavy metals, food pesticides, air pollution, electromagnetic stress, molds) to systemic (other co-infections and viruses, adrenal fatigue, thyroid issues, leaky gut, candida, genetic expression) to personal (grief, loss, trauma, overwork), the immune system may become overwhelmed and succumb to delayed yet full-blown Lyme disease expression.[43]

The larger picture that I talked about in the introduction to this book, chronic illnesses being generally under evaluated and undertreated in our mainstream medical system, is another layer of complication when trying to determine a chronic Lyme disease diagnosis. There just is no place in the usual, mainstream model of medicine to evaluate a patient with chronic, complex health issues who may have chronic Lyme disease.

The setup for modern patient care, with family doctors being the primary care and main access point into the system, does not work well for fully evaluating complex chronic illness.

There is not enough time per appointment to look at the whole picture, and the tools that the family physicians have at their disposal are geared for acute pathologies for which they tend to recommend drugs or surgery, not in-depth assessment of multi-faceted chronic conditions.

The family physician is set up to refer to other specialties, and there is not yet a specialty within the *conventional* health care system that holistically identifies and treats the root cause of chronic illness. But the role of the family physician can be very helpful to you in a number of different ways, even though they cannot likely diagnose or treat chronic Lyme disease.

Their access to various insured medical specialties can save you a lot of time, money and aggravation in at least ruling out what you may *not* have and doing some initial screening. I'll talk more about some specifics in Chapter Three to help you with this, so that you can know what you need to discuss with your physician.

When you do get to the point of narrowing in on a Lyme diagnosis, and beginning treatment via a Lyme specialist, your family doctor can be your ally when they are working as a team member in conjunction with your Lyme MD, in ways in which I'll also describe in Chapter Three.

So now what?

How do you as a typical health care consumer go about evaluating whether this is in fact chronic Lyme or some other type of chronic disease or syndrome? After all, you're not a doctor!

Who will help you assess this properly? Do you *really* have fibromyalgia, chronic fatigue syndrome, multiple sclerosis? How would you know? How far do you go in investigating this for yourself, and how? When do you just take the doctor's word for it, and when do you know to look further?

I'm going to do my best to give you some suggestions that you can consider to help you through this stressful dilemma. You've come this far. You're not happy with what you've been told. Your intuition is telling you there's something wrong, and you still don't have all the answers, in spite of what you've been told so far. You feel like there is more going on. Trust it.

Step 1: Why your starting place is self-education to learn more about Lyme Disease

I know it seems that the first place to start when you're sick is to go to your primary physician. But Lyme is different. For the reasons I've explained, taking that action if you do have Lyme, and expecting satisfying results will just lead you on a frustrating merry go round, as you've likely already found out with your current attempts at diagnosis and obtaining effective treatment.

First, you'll need to have a better idea about what Lyme disease is all about, so you can formulate the kinds of questions you need to answer in order to start figuring out your own situation.

This includes learning more about Lyme disease symptoms and those of common co-infections, and more about the professionals who diagnose them. You will need this information in order to be able to assess what type of professional is going to be able help you next, and what types cannot. You need to know this in order to start making some decisions about who you will consult with — to help you either get a Lyme diagnosis, or to confidently rule it out.

A well-rounded resource for starting your Lyme disease education is *The Canadian Lyme Disease Foundation* website, http://canlyme.com/. I'll be referring to this website at various sections of the book to suggest specific further reading.

Step 2: You will need to learn about how Lyme is tested, so you know that you are getting the best testing available.

This is important because if you're told by your family doctor, or other specialist, that you *don't* have Lyme because the test they did was negative (if they thought to test it at all), you will know that this may not be true. You may still have Lyme. You will need to know that *all* the available tests still have flaws, why the doctors interpreting the tests are not created equal, and why even lab tests are not the whole story in diagnosing Lyme.

Lyme disease testing: the good news and the bad news

Here's the bad news: *The Canadian Lyme Disease Foundation* website states *"There is no universally accepted test for Lyme disease. Every lab test has its advantages and disadvantages, but overall Lyme tests in Canada are largely flawed."* [44] So why bother testing, if there is no one test that is reliable in pinning down a Lyme diagnosis? If you decide to ask your doctor to test you anyway, what are the tests currently used to diagnose Lyme disease in Canada, and how do you access them?

Here's a brief, simplified summary of what is going on with Lyme testing, so that you can be informed when discussing this with your family physician or any further specialized practitioner.

In the province of Ontario, Canada where I live, the only tests (available via your family physician's orders, and fully funded by your provincial health care insurance,

OHIP) used to screen Lyme disease are called 1) the ELISA test and 2) the Western Blot test, which tests for only one of the many strains of the Lyme bacteria *Borrelia burgdorferi*.[45]

The second blood test is only done if the first is positive. *If the first test is negative, you will likely be told that you do not have Lyme disease.*

These tests, performed at the Public Health Ontario Laboratory, are based upon 1994 guidelines set by the USA-based CDC (Center for Disease Control) as recommended by the Canadian Public Health Laboratory Network, and approved by federal regulators in Health Canada.[46]

There are other, more sensitive Lyme lab tests available from a few specific laboratories in the USA that are not covered by OHIP. You can get access to this testing via a provincial Naturopathic physician you consult with, as one option. This also comes with some cautions, which I will outline in a moment. These US-based tests will not be ordered by your Canadian family physician, because they do not fall under the approved standards for medical practice in Canada.

Here are some of the key problems with the approved Lyme testing in Canada:[47, 48]

- The ELISA and Western Blot tests used in Ontario measure the immune system's response to only one strain of Borrelia burgdorferi. There are many more strains that could be present, yet are not tested. This can produce a false negative result, meaning that you can still have Lyme, but the test says you don't.

- The Western Blot measures the immune response to the infectious agent, not components of the agent itself, making it an indirect test.[49] There are various reasons why a compromised immune system cannot muster up enough response for the antibodies to show up in order to produce a positive result in testing, so the test ends up being deemed negative. Lyme bacteria are tricky to detect in their various forms and can evade an immune response. This can also produce a false negative test result.

• Of particular concern in acute Lyme disease testing is that your antibodies to Lyme, if you do produce them, may not show up until at least three weeks after being infected.[50] So a test which is done right around the time of a suspected or actual tick bite may be negative, and misleading. If you retest and Lyme antibodies show up later, this is already placing you past the window of time where you need to start treatment in order to prevent chronic Lyme disease.

• In order to diagnose Lyme, your physician may place his or her diagnostic decision solely on an initial, often unreliable lab test, instead of on clinical diagnosis. Lyme experts state that Lyme is primarily a clinical diagnosis. This means it's a decision made by the discerning doctor based on your history, physical, symptoms, and risk — not by a lab test alone. So no matter which lab tests are used, even if you use a more reliable or sensitive one, the diagnosis of Lyme disease still comes down to a Lyme-savvy doctor making a clinical assessment and utilizing professional judgment.

The good news is that there are tests that are generally considered to be more useful to augment your physician's clinical diagnostic decision. They are:

- A Western Blot that sends a report that visually displays its significant 'bands' (like a bar code) on the test report, corresponding to the likelihood of Lyme. The well-informed physician can then examine the report to make a more discerning judgment call, rather than relying on a computer at the lab using the narrower CDC guidelines for interpreting it, and in turn making certain judgments that can result in false negatives.[51, 52] In other words, reading the lab test report is also a grey, interpretive area. This type of test report is not available in Canada. More information about specific USA labs that do this testing, including those that test more than one strain of Borrelia burgdorferi, can be found at The Canadian Lyme Disease Foundation website: http://canlyme.com/just-diagnosed/testing/.

- Other specific lab tests that look at more indirect markers for Lyme can be ordered and evaluated by a Lyme Literate physician, to build a case further supporting a clinical diagnosis of Lyme.[53]

What does this mean for you, if you get a tick bite, a bull's-eye rash, onset of acute symptoms and suspect you have Lyme? It means that the physician you see, be it a family MD or Emergency MD, will need to be aware of Lyme, forgo lab testing for now (or do the insurance-covered testing, but not put diagnostic 'weight' on it, if it's negative), make a clinical diagnosis, and give you the correct type of antibiotics to treat it.

But even the currently used CDC/IDSA guidelines for the length of time that you need antibiotics are of concern.[54]

There are Lyme-literate physicians who believe that a two week course of oral antibiotics is not long enough to completely eradicate acute Lyme disease. Guidelines for physicians (based on ILADS recommendations) suggest at least 20 days of antibiotics.[55] Other well-respected guidelines for physicians suggest a longer, as in four to six week, course of antibiotics.[56] So even with treatment, you may risk a recurrence due to not treating it for long enough in the first place.

If your doctor relies on lab testing right away, it will very likely give a negative result, even if you do have Lyme, so they may not give you any antibiotics at all, or they may delay treating you for too long, risking that the disease could become chronic.

So, the conundrum:

Due to the current lab tests not providing a black and white *yes* or *no* with acute or chronic Lyme diagnosis, the only way that chronic Lyme disease can be accurately diagnosed is by seeing a Lyme literate physician. This expert spends enough time with you to thoroughly review your detailed history, and does other lab tests and a physical exam to either determine the strong possibility that you have Lyme, or to rule it out. Note: *'strong possibility'*.

The LLMD may still prefer to assume a working (or

tentative) diagnosis of Lyme, start treatment, evaluate your response — and then based on that response, finally be more confident that your chronic illness is indeed due to Lyme disease. The physician will also do careful evaluation for specific co-infections and viruses, which can play a significant role in your health picture as well.

Learn who you can rely on to identify chronic Lyme disease and how they do it

You will need to learn how to search for an appropriate Lyme-aware professional who you can trust, who can evaluate you using your detailed history, physical examination, lengthy interview, and testing. Where do you look, how do you pick this person, and how do you get in to see them?

Lyme Literate physicians

Finding a Lyme specialist (often abbreviated as LLMD or LLND, depending on whether their original training began as a medical doctor or as a naturopathic doctor) can be a daunting task. They are few in number, spread out in location, and tend to be expensive to consult.

These highly trained professionals have bravely gone off the beaten trail in medicine because for various reasons, they saw a need to help patients suffering with Lyme disease who were not being helped, and they found a way to do it. They have sought specialized training and shared insights and are willing to push the envelope of their profession. They tend to be tireless pioneers who really want to address the mess of misdiagnosis, and the needless suffering that affects increasing numbers of people due to the phenomenon of untreated Lyme disease.

Because their practice of diagnosing and treating Lyme may risk legal scrutiny, some Lyme literate physicians (who likely do not follow the IDSA/CDC overly narrow guidelines for practice) take a low-profile approach and can be accordingly hard to find. Here are a few ways that you can independently look for these physicians in order to access their medical expertise in diagnosing Lyme:

- Direct Internet searches for individual listings for Lyme Literate MD's or ND's.

- National Lyme Websites that may have local Lyme chapters with referral networks.

- Facebook groups where patients share their direct experience and resources.

- Blog talk online radio shows where various health care professionals interview experts in Lyme, or host their own Lyme information shows or webinars.

- Direct referral by a non-MD health care practitioner who sees lots of other patients with Lyme to help them with various health issues (eg. nutritionist), and who may refer you to an LLMD they are associated with. This is how I found the LLMD I now work with.

Where you will likely *not* find a specific Lyme Literate MD is via your family physician's referral network, especially in Ontario, Canada.

Hopefully, you will be supported in looking further if you choose to discuss this with your family MD. But more than likely, this will be a path you will need to take without your family physician's guidance. You may even find that they discourage you from looking further for diagnostic help. This could be due to their either being unaware about chronic Lyme, not having their professional association's encouragement to learn about its subtle diagnostic and treatment possibilities, or simply not having the time due to intense general practice demands.

The next step: How do you start sifting through this medical maze?

So you want to go ahead and find your path towards confirming or denying a Lyme diagnosis. This chapter has likely brought up even more questions than answers about how to proceed! How do you work with your own family doctor, on what kinds of preliminary testing and issues? What conventional specialist referrals do you go ahead with from your family doctor to rule in or out various other illnesses or diseases, and how do you interpret what that professional has told you, especially if they also are unaware of Lyme?

What do you need to figure out as you get started, and how do you decide what to do first in order to start getting more specific medical help and investigating whether you have Lyme or not? When do you stop going to more conventional medical specialists, and how do you figure out who to finally go and see, to end the doctor merry-go-round and get some real answers?

When do you strike out on your own, away from your family doctor's known territory and referral network, to pursue other resources — and what does that even mean? What about insurance issues, figuring out what is covered and what isn't? How do you get around that?

In Chapter Two, I'll tell you my own story, include what worked and didn't work for me on my long and complicated path to chronic Lyme disease diagnosis. I hope that knowing my story will give you some valuable insight in order to save you significant time, money, aggravation and suffering. And then in Chapter Three, we'll get into some insight on how to navigate the medical system to proceed on your own diagnostic journey, so you can get going to solve your own medical mystery once and for all.

Chapter 2: My 30-year Journey
Looking for Answers Before Getting My Lyme Diagnosis

"People with chronic illness are some of the strongest people I know."

— *Dr. Jess Armine* [57]

"When crisis comes up, surrender to it. Let it take you on the ride of your life, because it will."

— *Panache Desai* [58]

"Surrender to the inability to surrender. And that opens the door."

— *Peggy Kornegger* [59]

Have you noticed that although you *thought you knew* how your life was going to turn out, the Universe seemed to have other plans for you?

When my husband Jeff and I happily and optimistically got together at age 33, and then married at 35, we had no way of knowing that most of our efforts, financial resources and attention from that day forward would be spent on chasing answers for my ongoing health challenges.

As an ambitious, career-centered woman in my 20's,

I didn't realize how much of the next 35 years would be spent trying to find my way through multiple mysterious illness episodes, where each time I thought this was surely the final one — that I was really going to be OK now. That this particular label, this new strategy, this skilled professional, or this innovative treatment was *finally* going to be the one to do it — this was the one that was going to get me well.

Every time Jeff and I thought that we'd finally cracked the code on my diagnosis, and had a new direction of health care undertaken, we would find that yet another round of illness was lurking around the corner. Our daily efforts would be spent denying and excusing what was happening, having brief respites where it all seemed to be improving, and then the familiar decline would inevitably happen again. This pattern would repeat itself for over three decades.

Years were spent trying to "make do" with my drastically limited energy. I would push myself just to function daily. I selected an endless, painstaking parade of new work schedules, over several careers, and created and recreated several business incarnations, always looking for a new way to manage my life while living with unexplained, profound fatigue and significant, multi-systemic symptoms.

With every change, every new approach, every fresh start, I told myself that these external changes, these intense internal attempts to better myself and improve my attitudes and thinking, or these new, even more fulfilling careers or business start-ups, would be my ticket to a vibrant life and good health.

I was wrong.

Critical to journeying my way out of this whole mess, was finally learning that these decades of illness in fact had a name and a key reason for occurring: chronic Lyme disease, along with several co-infections, caused by an undetected tick bite — likely in my 20's. Added to that mix was a whole bunch of physical and emotional stressors, some in my youth, some lifelong habits, and even the reality of dealing with unexplained severe chronic illness fed that negative spiral. It all added up to a major assault on my immune system's ability to handle all of these foreign invaders.

My story has parallels to countless other people who are finally diagnosed with chronic Lyme disease after many years of health struggles.

It's my hope that by recounting my experience, you'll be able to recognize similar elements in your own life. Through examination and reflection of what I've done and not done, learned and wished I'd learned, I hope that you will be able to make informed choices that will create a new path for your own life — one that brings you swift and satisfying recovery of your health.

My health challenges started at a young age

When I was in my mid-20's, I decided to go for counseling. I had gone through many challenges already, although I thought at the time these were solely related to growing up with a mother with mental illness, a father who was emotionally absent, their separation on the day they dropped me off at University, and the fallout of being forced to be emotionally independent from a very young age because of all of these dysfunctions.

I didn't realize, until much later in life, that a series of childhood illnesses — so severe at times that I missed anything from months at a time to almost a full year of primary school — had also created the perfect storm to stress my immune system to the point of being high risk for whatever else came along. I had years of chronic ear infections, a tonsillectomy with incomplete anesthesia that created PTSD, a mysterious round of vertigo which lasted for months, as well as a year of severe headaches requiring investigation for a brain tumor (there wasn't one). Add to that significant digestive issues, undiagnosed stomach pain that had me living on antacids for years, a few rounds of pneumonia in high school, and severe flu, sinus infection, and bronchitis several times a year for most of my life. I was anxious, depressed at times, and frequently felt alone and scared. But there was no perceived significance about all of this in my conscious awareness. I just felt what I felt. Sometimes I wondered what was wrong with me that made me so unhappy so often.

I thought it was 'normal' to have mom sick in bed (again) with the bedroom door closed (again) — for days or weeks at a time. I thought it was 'normal' to tiptoe–literally and figuratively — around the house, preparing for the inevitable emotional fireworks that could be innocently elicited from her at any given time. I didn't know that the way I was treated and manipulated by her, largely due to her own state of overwhelm and undiagnosed and untreated mental and physical health issues, would now be classed as emotional abuse. From living with my mom, I honed my considerable lifelong skills at perceiving someone's subtle emotional nuances. I figured if I knew how to judge what I needed to do or say, I could sometimes avoid provoking her and being the target of yet another painful emotional outburst. But I also learned that usually my efforts were not good enough. The angry outbursts occurred anyway.

Into my 20's

I soldiered on, as all children do, compensating the best I could. I was a 'good girl', studying hard and getting good marks at school. I did what I was told. Books were my solace. I realized, as I grew older, that achievement and hard work was always my distraction to make me feel that I had some kind of value in the world. It was also my ticket out of the house: high enough marks for admission to the limited-enrolment, four-year university program of my choice, Occupational Therapy at the University of Western Ontario, in 1973.

My health problems continued, but stayed in the realm of what I considered more minor and unrelated ones at University and in my early 20's: colds, flu's, sinus infections, yeast infections, seasonal depression, digestive issues, anxiety. I just thought this backdrop was normal. My awareness of what healthy foods and a balanced life-style actually consisted of was pretty sketchy back then. I partied hard during university, barely passing my first year, but then became a serious student by my 4th year. By then, I realized that I was soon going to be let loose on the world as a practicing Occupational Therapist. I had better know what I was doing!

I got my first job at University Hospital in London, Ontario. It was fabulous. I loved the teaching hospital atmosphere, and the various areas I was able to work in (orthopedics, stroke and spinal cord rehab, rheumatic diseases). After a few years, I specialized in rehabilitation of traumatic hand injuries, where I stayed for the rest of my nine years there. I worked with hand cases until age 33, advancing to supervisory and specialty positions. I was even able to teach at the university I had attended, travel to do workshops and conference presentations on hand splinting and rehab for therapists, and constantly be involved in continuing education. I worked overtime a lot, and was enthusiastically immersed in my role.

During that time, I began to have increasing and distressing health issues. I didn't really make any connection between this and my tendency to overwork, overplay, and overachieve, while still carrying with me the scars from my childhood. Those were as yet still largely unconscious, but they made me secretly feel I wasn't good enough, and would more insistently take their toll on my body. As I felt worse, I just pushed harder. I just denied more.

My first significant time period off work for illness happened when I was 28. At the time, I was diagnosed by my family physician as having Epstein Barr virus, 'burnout' or 'yuppie flu' as this chronic fatigue-type illness was called back then in the popular press. I was off work for two whole months with exhaustion, low fever, and mild achiness. Despite my critical colleagues who accused me behind my back of 'faking it' to get the summer off (or so it was admitted to me later), I really felt lousy and slept a lot.

I had no way of knowing at the time that this was merely the first episode of what was to be so many more occurrences in the coming years, which is a common pattern in those of us with chronic, invisible illness of unknown cause. But it was my first taste of the horrible, secret feeling that went with it: shame. What was wrong with me? Why was I so tired? Why didn't any amount of self-pushing seem to make me be able to get up and get going? Why was I so flawed as to have this non-existent, silly illness that was the brunt of social and media jokes?

Into my 30's

But I did recover, I did go back to work, and I thought that was all behind me. I got married at age 30, was advancing in my occupational therapy career, and thought that all was well for a time, at least. As my fatigue increased, I would just compensate by sleeping more on the weekends — and pushing harder all week.

By age 32, crisis would hit again. My mom committed suicide. My new marriage crumbled. I was co-executor of my mom's estate with my sister, who lived 3,000 kms away, and that meant I would have to be in charge of dealing with the sorting and selling of mom's house and her 30 years of possessions. She had three tenants in her house who had to be legally evicted, one of whom was violent. My sister's overbearing partner was terrified that I would do anything that may waste a dime that they would inherit, and so I was under massive scrutiny for every tiny decision I might make. This was pre-internet days, so everything had to be physically couriered back and forth to my sister and her partner, for co-signature after co-signature, arranged by excruciating phone call after phone call. I thought I would burst with the stress of all of it. Then add to this heap my unsupportive (former) husband who decided I was not being much fun anymore, who withdrew completely in a sulk.

I pretty much felt I was losing it most days. The therapists around me at work kept to themselves, and gave me a wide berth. I used up all my break times making endless phone arrangements. I became more and more isolated, alone and exhausted. I moved out of my home and legally separated from my first husband. I lost what I had thought were 'true' friendships because I was not available to be a friend. I was raw, numb and unable to reach out for help. I just tried to keep my head up and do the next task. I didn't see any way for things to be different.

Kindness, and extensive physical help, from two old family friends, Joan and Al Shaw, and from my cherished Aunt Alice and Uncle Jack, somehow got me through the worst of this time. Or so I thought. I was also lucky enough to develop a new relationship, which was with my eventual second husband, Jeff, while we were both in the raw stages of our respective marital separations. We talked for hours and hours and we held each other up. Against all odds we may have had from the fact of being a 'rebound' relationship, we have been solidly together since that time.

My health, however, was not so solid. The stresses of that time frame, and more to come, were mounting — and my body was keeping score. By age 33, about a year after I moved to Sarnia to live with Jeff, and while trying to keep up with commuting the resulting 110 km to my job in London, I suffered from debilitating fatigue again. I kept pushing to keep going, again. I was able to adjust some of my work hours and even work at home one day a week, writing a professional journal article I was working on for publication, but it just wasn't enough. By September of that year, I had to go off work on what turned out to be long-term disability, and then a few years later, hand in my resignation.

This time, we looked further and deeper for answers, a quest that led us over the next couple of years to various physicians — specialists in many disciplines — within a 500 km radius. My diagnosis at this point, again popular in the press at the time, was Chronic Fatigue Syndrome. The treatment consisted of rest and lifestyle management to conserve my limited energy as best I could. I also was found to have hypothyroidism and started on new medication for that. I saw a regional specialist to be evaluated for Lyme disease, on the urging of a local acquaintance, but was told I had a parasite — not Lyme disease — and was treated for the parasite.

On the urging of my Aunt Alice, I also sought the assessment of a Doctor of Chinese medicine and Acupuncture, Professor Cedric Cheung. Traveling over an hour each way, three times a week, for acupuncture treatments and taking Chinese herbs, I was starting to improve. I was so fascinated by this whole process that I made a life-changing decision. I enrolled in Prof. Cheung's four-year program to study Chinese Medicine and Acupuncture, and formally resigned from my occupational therapy position around the same time.

We used up my retirement savings to pay my yearly tuition, and somehow I attended classes part time, while still ill and in bed a lot, and I studied full time. I continued to improve each year, and by my fourth year, was able to complete the clinical training hours and rigorous exams to graduate on time.

Into my 40's

Remarkably, I seemed to have those awful years of illness behind me and to have found the answer to my mysterious health problems. I proceeded to set up my own successful clinic with two employees, and quickly had a booming practice in Chinese Medicine complete with a waiting list. I embarked on a massive continuing education path, including a challenging specialty certificate in Chinese Medicine gynecology, from a well-known teacher in Colorado.

I was back! I was on! I worked hard for several years. Sure, I was so tired by Thursday evenings that I had anxiety attacks about trying to make it to work on Fridays. Sure, I worried constantly if I was a good enough practitioner — and felt huge anxiety about doing a good enough job to help so many desperate patients. It was 'normal' to pretty much collapse and need to rest and sleep most of the weekends, because I was so busy all week, right? I missed most of my two nephews' lives growing up because every weekend I would say, "Maybe next weekend I'll have enough energy to have them here for a visit". When my husband, who worked twelve hour shifts as a lab technician at Imperial

Oil, finally had a weekend off where we could have a fun getaway, I mostly slept.

After about seven years in my business, I finally had to face that I was too exhausted to continue this way. I made the drastic move to downsize my office, letting my staff go and reducing my hours. I was barely meeting my expenses and no longer paying myself, but kept hoping things would somehow get better. Not able to keep up on my own, I did go on to hire a wonderful student part-time to help with reception and office tasks for a couple of years.

More personal stresses mounted up within an intense time period starting in the late 90's. These included the sudden death of my dad (whom I had finally developed a closer relationship with as an adult) and a multitude of trips 3,000 km to British Columbia to clean out his house and belongings, along with my sister. There was a very painful breakup and betrayal with a close friend and business partner of some years. There was the declining health of Jeff's parents and eventual death of Jeff's dad; his mom's kidney failure, dialysis and subsequent kidney transplant; and even the death of our beloved family dog following a prolonged illness that had required intense physical caretaking.

Jeff and I, although we had not married until age 35, and in spite of experiencing some of my considerable health challenges right away, were still hoping to have a baby. But after several years of not conceiving, we concluded that we may be dealing with infertility. The few medical investigations we did toward that end were inconclusive. I continued to pee on pregnancy test sticks, month after month, holding my breath and waiting for a positive line — and then have yet another cry. That deep sadness, that I mostly kept private, was a constant strain too. I found myself avoiding friends and family with babies and young children, as it was always a painful reminder of our own childlessness. I just kept focusing on work and hoped somehow that this deep emotional pain would lessen. I would repeatedly dream about finally holding my own baby, but then wake up to an empty bed.

During this time I was also in the role of power of attorney for my beloved aunt and uncle, which required regular attention, during their collective years of health decline including her dementia. My uncle's death, and that of my aunt a few years later, represented a big loss for me. As you'll recall, they had been my close family since I was in my mid-20s. The distance I felt from my only sister, who lived so far away and had increasingly severe health and functional challenges with her diagnosis of multiple sclerosis, also weighed heavily on me.

During all these years, I consistently stepped up my holistic health care regime. I further cleaned up my diet, and sought out the help of counseling, physiotherapy, massage therapy, Naturopathic doctors, Chinese medicine, homeopathy, and chiropractic care. I saw my family doctor for regular blood screening and thyroid monitoring. I went to a gym and worked with an excellent trainer doing regular workouts for years, stopping only occasionally when I seemed to be injured, ill or too exhausted and couldn't modify my program to accommodate these things. I saw a gynecologist for bio-identical hormone replacement therapy when I entered perimenopause and had hot flashes so severe that I was awake every half hour with drenching sweats. I meditated, read natural diet books, and loaded up on self help books. The various, and often vague diagnoses I received (and assumed to be true) included hypothyroidism, chronic fatigue syndrome, hormonal issues, and sudden joint and muscle pain syndromes that seemed to come out of the blue. The pattern of intermittent flus, colds and sinus infections continued, as did the unrelenting fatigue.

I also constantly re-evaluated my life, how I lived, what I thought about, who I spent time with, and how I could continue to better myself. Still, the unrelenting fatigue episodes would flatten me and that would influence every decision I made and everything I did, trying in vain to compensate for it, live in spite of it, and start to treat it.

By 2000, as I was going through some of the personal grief, stresses and even downsizing my Chinese Medicine career, I embarked on yet another parallel direction. I decided that I wanted to give my intuitive side more support and exploration. Maybe that would open up new avenues for me, provide me with a renewed feeling of energy, and give me new answers to my health. I told myself that maybe I just wasn't cut out for running a Chinese medicine practice after all, even though I loved supporting the health and well-being of my long-term patients, loved the work and found it very rewarding.

So I excitedly found that Lori Wilson, founder of Inner Access 101, taught a unique range of intuitive exploration classes. I took every course that she offered, and embarked on what was to be a new and spiritually rich phase of my life. I learned how to guide clients through past life regression exploration. I developed an ability to channel a special spirit guide for life guidance and support that continues to this day. I learned how to practice medical intuition, to receive detailed information from the body to help people with their health care decisions and mind-body connections. I formally trained with Inner Access 101 to teach these programs, and also developed a new one that I taught to participants as part of a vacation retreat package. I loved it all. I had renewed hope, too, that applying this new set of skills and business focus — activating what felt like a true calling — would be the way in which I would finally feel well.

I further reduced the size of my Chinese medicine practice, and incorporated these other new intuitive areas into my work, again with success and happy clients. This new work seemed to really agree with me, and I decided that it was time to make a choice in my career and business focus. Maybe the reason I was still having health and energy issues was because I just needed a change of career and had to eliminate the challenges of a demanding patient health care practice.

Into my 50's

By 2004, with mixed feelings, I closed my Chinese medicine practice altogether, deciding to work from home doing ad hoc teaching in various locations, workshops and 1:1 client appointments, hoping that in this way, I would be able to regain more energy and greater life balance.

For the next five years, I worked out of my home office doing sporadic intuitive work, with weeks of reduced hours and resting in between. The only problem was — although it appeared to the outside world that I had a successful business, financially I was barely breaking even — covering only my office expenses and some of my continuing education. I couldn't work enough hours to afford to pay myself. I kept hoping this, too, would be temporary. I thought I was mostly doing OK health-wise, but I realize in retrospect that I had just become accustomed to constantly compensating for my limitations, while looking OK enough to the outside world (with effort, of course) as I was well-versed in pretending I was fine to myself and others. That continual thread of shame for not coping with a 'normal' schedule, feeling lousy despite supposedly having nothing really wrong with me, continued to haunt me.

I constantly thought of ways that I could use all of my skills, while working from a home office with limited, tightly structured hours. I kept pushing myself to learn more, and be better, hoping I would finally be good enough at something if I worked hard enough and took yet another course. Again, my choices were mostly driven by my health reality and influenced by my inner angst, but my level of awareness about this continued to be below my active, conscious radar. I just kept looking for cool, challenging, stimulating things to do and learn, that were in helping professions, which would give me greater flexibility of time and lifestyle.

In 2007-8 I become a life coach, obtaining Power Coaching® certifications for both one on one and group coaching from Coaching and Leadership International Inc. in British Columbia. This I loved as well. Buoyed by renewed enthusiasm, I proceeded to buy new furniture and set up an office for my new coaching practice in a holistic healing centre. Here, I actually combined Chinese medicine, individual and group Power Coaching® programs, and intuitive services. I kept up with continuing education in the coaching world, and began to do a series of business mastermind groups and take small business development training.

Again, I told myself I was 'back', I was OK, and *finally this time I was really going to make a go of it*, business wise and health-wise. I dove into a high-level business Mastermind group that was a huge financial investment. Jeff and I were so thrilled that I seemed to be doing better now, and I was ready to increase my hours and make this a big success. I then decided to close my latest in-person client office, and began offering a unique blend of my group coaching skills in a home-based, phone and internet-delivered business model. The first few months of the Mastermind group were going great, and I was devouring the stimulating learning material as well as the camaraderie and support of the group. But even this brief health respite was rudely interrupted.

Jeff and I had gone to our treasured vacation spot in Cuba in February 2009, and both of us got very ill. Jeff contracted an acute food and then blood poisoning, rendering him almost unconscious, and ultimately requiring emergency hospitalization and treatment. Fortunately, he began to recover within a few days, but it was a very frightening time. A few days further into that fateful vacation, I got a knock-down flu with a high fever, sweats, exhaustion, and unbearable stomach pain. Upon returning home, and still having significant problems, I obtained a referral to a gastroenterologist, was diagnosed as having inflammation in my stomach as well as esophageal spasms of unknown origin, and took acid-reducing medication for over a year. My energy had declined again as well. I figured I could just compensate more again and it would hopefully get better.

I continued with the mastermind group, and eager business planning, over the next few months. That October, I attended a live three-day event for the Mastermind group in Maui, which Jeff and I combined with an amazing vacation. It was fabulous. We were so optimistic.

There was just one teensy problem. I was getting much worse again, health-wise. By that fall, I started having acute abdominal pain that kept me awake at night and I took Tylenol every night to try to manage to get some sleep. My energy level was declining. I was getting a bit depressed, even though I loved the way my business planning was going. I was having more muscle pain. I was getting some more brain fog. I shrugged it all off as just being the approach of winter with being busier with this exciting work planning. I suffered from S.A.D. (seasonal affective disorder/depression) every winter, so as usual, I told myself I would just stay on St. John's Wort for another year, and use my lamp that simulates sunlight every morning. I booked an appointment to see my Naturopath to review my huge list of supplements. *No sweat!*

I decided to hire one of my Mastermind members, who

I felt was a huge resource, because she had cured herself and her husband of stage four cancers. She was very knowledgeable in holistic health, and so I asked her to assess me so we could see what might be going on. It took all the courage I could muster up to even admit I was having problems again. My current health professionals had nothing new to offer me. Why not try a new approach?

My list of possible problems, which were confirmed with further testing of stool samples, urine and blood screening: high levels of mercury toxicity, candida, leaky gut, adrenal fatigue, and food sensitivities. All of these factors were collectively creating a pile of adverse symptoms that could explain so much of my history, all of which had seemed unrelated. I received a new level of education in holistic health, filling in gaps in areas that I had heard about in my health travels and reading over the years, but had not realized they applied to me.

We revamped my supplement program, and I did some rounds of mercury detoxing via a medical doctor whom I was able to work with on the phone and online. It did not go well. Despite conscientious care from my colleague, I had very rough reactions to my dietary changes and to the detoxing itself, with a lot of adverse symptoms and a rapid decline. I became very depressed that winter, to the point of feeling suicidal at times. Only my husband and a few close friends even heard about my renewed struggling. We assumed that it was part of the healing phase, and decided I just needed to ride it out—in the hopes that my body would detox more completely and I would improve. We hoped that this time we were getting at the root of my health issues.

I kept going with the mastermind program, but by February had to withdraw and did not finish the last two months. I gave up my business plans, and stopped marketing my planned new group coaching program. I withdrew from business and my life. I just slipped off the business scene again with a sense of shame and deep despair that I couldn't keep up due to these vague maladies, which seemed off the medical mainstream's radar.

We heard about an outpatient clinic in Arizona that primarily was a cancer clinic but also treated patients holistically for issues like my leaky gut. With my practitioner's recommendation, we contacted the clinic and decided to go to Arizona for a few weeks starting in April 2010 to explore treatment. Maybe this green juice fasting, colonics, raw food diet, infrared saunas, and so on would finally work, and I could continue with my mercury detoxing program and heal my gut. Upon liquidating our retirement savings, Jeff obtaining a leave from work, and even our dog and cats having been taken in temporarily by close friends — we flew to Arizona. That three-week adventure turned into three months and wiped out a good chunk of our retirement savings. We had to remortgage our house when we got home to cover the $90,000 in expenses on our maxed out credit cards.

I kept hoping that this was the path to getting well, but in Arizona I got so ill and my liver enzymes became so elevated that the clinic doctor thought I may have a serious liver disease. I was too ill to leave. My weight went down to what it had been in pre-adolescence, and I became weaker and even more depressed. I could hardly leave my recliner, where I spent every day at the clinic, on various endless antioxidant and other intravenous infusions, all of which were designed to boost my immune system to help me get well again. At the end of each day we would go back to our crappy little motel room, where I would crawl under four blankets (in typically hot Arizona weather), too weak and brain fogged to even read or watch TV most of those evenings.

During the latter part of our stay in Arizona, Jeff's mom had surgery for bladder cancer and had such severe complications in her recovery that she was in critical care. Jeff's two sisters lived in the same city as the hospital where their mother was, and were keeping vigil, and they had to inform him that she had decided to discontinue all life sustaining options. His younger sister was very upset with Jeff for his refusal to leave me in Arizona and fly home immediately. We both wanted to get home as soon as possible. My doctor told me I needed to stay. I was too sick for Jeff to leave me on my own, yet his mom was facing imminent death. After almost a week of this tension, and with my medical doctor's caution to keep my blood work monitored closely and have some local medical follow-up arranged, we flew home near the end of June 2010.

The trip home was a grief, exhaustion and illness-filled blur for me, as was my trying to cope when I got home. Within fifteen minutes of us arriving home late one evening, Jeff drove over an hour to his mom's hospital. He continued to spend as much time as possible there in the coming days. I was barely able to move around and stand up much at home, and I needed help to take care of myself.

With the blur of this crisis with Jeff's mom, we all just tried to manage as best we could for the next ten difficult days up until her death, and then to somehow get through the funeral. I was never well enough to make the trip to see her before she died, and that continues to be a source of grief and guilt. I also felt shame and more guilt for the fact that I couldn't muster up more stamina despite making huge efforts. Indeed, I just kept hoping I wouldn't faint in front of everyone and even feared being seen as shamefully disruptive or distracting as I tried to manage through the visitation and the funeral.

The next few years were a time of constant health care focus. I went to see a Naturopathic physician (ND) in another city three times weekly. I had to get help for rides when my husband was working because I was too weak, ill and brain — fogged to drive myself. The ND did ongoing testing and treatment with anti-oxidant IV infusions and extensive supplements. This was considered to be the best treatment for my diagnosis of mercury (and other heavy metals) toxicity as well as toxicity of multiple petrochemicals. We didn't know why or how this toxicity had occurred, but were led to believe it was at the root of my problems nonetheless.

I gradually phased off the raw food and juicing diet that had been one of the mainstays of treatment in Arizona, but my energy level and ability to function through day to day activity took a long time to improve. My daily routine was highly structured and packed with various holistic and energetic methods of treatment, lots of professional appointments, and a labor-intensive yet impeccable whole-foods diet.

Jeff and I will be eternally grateful for our close, long-standing friends and their kind vigilance and caring during that time. Our friend Joan, an occupational therapist whom I had first met at University, came to stay with us for days at a time to help us out. We so appreciated her kindness and generosity. *She just got it.* She did whatever needed to be done. She dove into my extensive meal prep and my restricted dietary needs, stocked our freezer with delicious meals, helped out with the animals, supported me around my health care routine as well as my volatile state of mind, and just loved us in her quiet and powerful way.

In order to keep up with our monthly bills, which amounted to over $3,000 in health care alone, my husband began working extensive overtime hours. Tension in the house was often high, due to both of us being so exhausted, let alone so worn down by so many years of recurrent illness. Our "recreation" consisted of watching an occasional movie together, which was truthfully often planned ahead and then cancelled several times, ordinarily due to Jeff being called in for overtime yet again, and his feeling he couldn't turn it down.

This spirit-sucking lifestyle would continue for what felt like an eternity. In fact, the worst of this particular health decline lasted about another year and a half. We stopped booking anything to do socially, because I felt too ill trying to manage myself and the entire household including our three pets, and of course in order to keep up with the financials, Jeff would go to work at a moment's notice. We felt we just had to keep going like this, in the hopes that eventually I would detox enough to get better again. During this time I was so grateful for my health care professionals who were compassionate and caring, as they were my only source of socialization with the outside world, sometimes for weeks on end.

We rarely had contact with friends or family. Occasionally, one of our close friends would invite us over for dinner, but she was dealing with a severe health crisis of her own. Therefore I felt guilty not being able to support her more myself. I again concluded, as I did at so many other times of long-term illness, that this was my reality of living with chronic illness. I was alone, people have busy lives, and if you can't show up to join in to their world, you don't exist.

So Jeff and I just forged on, mostly by staying on 'survival mode' in every way. At the times that I could manage to stick my head above water — and come out of my numb, depressed, ill, exhausted state — I was emotionally volatile. In fact, I was alternatively grateful beyond all words for Jeff's unwavering support and stamina, yet angry at the world for my fate, angry at Jeff for always going to work, but financially desperate for him to do so. Threading through every waking moment were feelings of profound guilt and shame for being so dependent on him in every way in order to manage my pathetic life. There were many times that I became suicidal. I begged him to please divorce me, so that he could create a new life for himself, one without carrying the burden of me and my illness. He refused to leave and just hugged me, saying, "We'll get through this." I often thought, "This man deserves a medal". I felt I didn't deserve *him*.

Finally, by the fall of 2012, I was improving again. In fact, I was beginning to have hope again. I thought that with careful planning, I could return to working even one day a week. I took on one long-term phone coaching and intuitive work client. I decided to return to a very small clinical practice, one combining Chinese Medicine, acupuncture and Power Coaching®. In January 2013, I rented a furnished treatment room one day a week in a local holistic health centre, and took on my first few clients.

I was able to cautiously expand that to two days a week within another six months. I was back! I was working again! Sure, that was all I could do, but it was worth it! I felt like a real human being again, back out in the world, making enough money to pay my rent, and pay for treatment supplies and toner for my printer! Sure, I couldn't afford to pay myself, but surely that would change soon, right? I had to have an hour nap at lunchtime to drag myself through a 10-5 day, do nothing on my days off other than manage the household, and I still had barely any energy to see another human being socially–but that would improve, right?

I reentered the world of mastermind and business coaching, eagerly drinking up and implementing my coach's helpful suggestions, and gradually re-organizing my practice, services and scheduling so that I was actually able to pay myself $500 a month. This was heaven. I was so optimistic, salivating at the prospects of getting back to the workforce again, making a difference in my clients' lives, contributing at home, and turning my life around, *finally*.

At the end of 2012, I took another step. I decided to increase my work to three days a week, and to contain it all to my rental office so that I could create better balance and boundaries between home and work. This was part of my larger plan, to start to have a real life again. I hoped that this would prevent the 'bleeding out' of work activities into all hours of the day and evening at home and hoped it would be the solution to creating some semblance of a normal life again. That's what I must need... *Better scheduling!* Better time management and priority setting! Even better organization than I was already doing! That would *surely* make me have a life again!

There was only one teensy problem...again. My health and energy were severely declining. As clients dropped off, I made no effort to market for new ones. I didn't follow up with leads. I would breathe a sigh of relief when a client appointment was cancelled and I would take a nap instead. I was back down to only a few clients, my expenses were more than my income again, and I was...*relieved.* I realized that I had again been on that merry-go-round of pushing, striving, wishing and doing — and this time I accepted that my body simply could not keep up.

In February of 2013, I went through a six-week period of acute sciatica that came out of the blue. The pain was incapacitating. I had to cancel the remaining few clients I had, did not make it into the office, and did what I could with phone appointments when I could sit up long enough. To say I was upset by this is a gross understatement. Knowing what I know now, I imagine that this was yet another manifestation of neurological chronic Lyme disease, which occurred acutely as I was getting more and more run down. At the time, it was seen as yet another bad luck, random occurrence.

As the sciatica gradually improved, with intensive treatment, I returned to seeing a few clients at work. For the rest of the year, there were weeks that I didn't show up at the office at all. I had only a small handful of clients. I made no efforts at building my business. It was all I could do to show up for the clients I had, care for them and treat them well, and slink home again. I faked it and smiled to the world, pretending that I was fine. I faked it to myself, hoping that it was not true, that this was not yet another unexplained decline with this weird assortment of toxins and chronic fatigue syndrome that barely felt like a real thing — and certainly was not seen as real in the eyes of mainstream medicine.

A key occurrence around this time was the introduction of provincial legislation regulating the practice of Chinese Medicine and Acupuncture in Ontario, effective April 1, 2013. This meant that I would now have to work full time hours in order to qualify to practice, as well as submitting an extensive application, preparing for and writing some qualifying exams. Practitioners failing to do this could find themselves assessed a $25,000 fine or even face imprisonment. I had to face the reality of the situation: I was 58 years old, getting more ill again with a mysterious ailment with no known cure. I was only able to work a few hours a week, and too exhausted to prepare for or do the exams, let alone figure out how I could sustain at least 20 Chinese medicine patient visits a week, on top of my desire to still maintain a coaching and intuitive services business. I dearly loved practicing all of these professional services. I now had to choose what would be feasible, based on my health.

On December 31, 2013, I terminated the lease on my 4th office rental. With a very heavy heart, I sadly packed up my office contents, took my proud array of professional certificates off the walls, and put them back into cardboard boxes. We moved my furniture home to store it in our basement, again. I put my furniture up for sale. Again.

My sister-in-law stung me that December with an unknowing remark, not ever understanding how much I had struggled with my health for so many decades and that I again had to give up my treasured work. When I told her I had some office cabinets for sale, knowing she might want them, she retorted, "Geez, I've never seen anybody go through buying and selling office furniture like you do!" With gritted teeth and hot tears in my eyes, I mumbled, 'I'm not feeling well enough to work. I had to close my office again." My remark was met with terse silence and a brisk change of subject. I concluded, yet again, that I was shameful: perhaps I was seen as a fraud, a faker, or at the very least, no one wanted to even acknowledge this weird set of chronic complaints that I persistently seemed to have.

During the last few months before I closed my office in 2013, in my renewed desperation for answers to my health, I began an online search in earnest. This was really the first time that I had fervently pursued anything and everything I could get my hands on. I don't know what flipped that switch, but it was an abrupt change in my attitude. It was a shift from continuing to trust or take referrals from my existing health care team, to realizing I again needed to look much further for information to my health dilemma.

I took a fresh look at all my symptoms. I signed up for every online holistic, functional and integrative medicine health summit I could find. I searched diverse topics and 'usual suspects' that I knew could underlie chronic illness: adrenal fatigue, hormonal and thyroid issues, gut issues including leaky gut, gluten and other food sensitivities; immune system issues, toxicity, MTHFR and other genetic issues, mental health issues, various dietary approaches to better health, and brain and nervous system issues. You name it, I attended it, bought the series, took notes, listened and wondered. I was not going to stop this time until I found *the answer!* I was no longer going to rely on thinking that my health care team members, as accomplished as they were, would *really think and wonder about my case the way it needed to be carefully thought about.* I was now determined to be the general contractor of my own health.

This turned out to be the best decision I had ever made.

Surviving the BIG FLU…sort of

In March of 2014, Jeff and I had a rare day off together. We were going for a short morning drive to get me out of the house for a break, after yet another twelve-day stretch of his constant working eight and twelve hour shifts. During this time he, as usual, also scrambled to do the grocery shopping, errands, household chores and some evening meals on the occasional day when he was home to eat. I took care of the animals, organized our daily tasks, planned and made most of our healthy meals, and struggled to keep up with the myriad tasks and appointments involved in my extensive health care regime. This scarce day off translated into a rare opportunity to get back onto the same page as a couple, as you will see later in this chapter.

During these early months of 2014 I was so grateful to be working even a little. I had maintained one intensive long-term coaching/intuitive services phone client whom I adored working with, along with doing occasional ad hoc appointments with other clients. I kept hoping to be able to expand my coaching business again one day, but mostly I was just hanging on by a thread.

We had just come through a particularly trying few months. I had a big detour just before Christmas of 2014 that almost finished me off. I developed a sudden onset of what I assumed was the flu on December 18, 2014. It was a somewhat typical malaise, replete with sore throat, exhaustion, body pain, high fever, chills and sweats. It was brutal. By Dec. 23, we called an ambulance, because I could barely breathe and was so weak and lightheaded that I needed help to get back and forth to the bathroom. I was too ill to travel to the hospital in the car, even to be able to sit up once I arrived in the emergency room. I had already fainted onto the bathroom floor once during the second night (and missed hitting my head on the shower stall by about an inch). My blood pressure was, at times, falling to 60/40. I felt like I was going to die. The ambulance attendants checked me out, but my chest was clear, my fever was only 102 degrees, and my oxygen levels tested OK. We decided not to go to emerg because I was not dehydrated and they assured me that there was really nothing other than IV hydration that they could do for the flu.

I continued like this for weeks, barely improving, even

once the fever went down. I have never been so weak in my life. It took almost a year to even begin to approach my pre-flu levels of function that I had achieved in 2014.

My portfolio of symptoms, which had occurred in various combinations and intensity over the years, had become even more extensive. As a baseline, I felt like I had a cross between a constant hangover, the flu, and as if I had just run 5 miles while out of shape. My muscles ached, and I had joint pain and stiffness in various places that came and went for no apparent reason. My brain fog, memory issues and cognitive challenges made it hard to concentrate—to the point where at times I would stand at the kitchen counter with a glass in my hand to get water, and forget what I was doing or what the glass was for.

My sensitivity to noise, smells, lights and social stimulation of any kind made it hard to go anywhere, or do much, without feeling overwhelmed. I was anxious and overwhelmed by everything. I had heart palpitations, and my blood pressure would dip to very low levels at times, making my constant dizziness and off-balance feeling even worse, sometimes to the point of feeling I would faint. Occasionally, the dizziness would become full-blown vertigo, along with occasional ear pain and pressure. I had odd visual disturbances and my eyes would just get too tired to focus properly. My digestive system produced one issue after the other on top of constant bloating. I couldn't trace what digestive issue was coming from where, despite my constant attention to diet and doing various extensive food sensitivity elimination diets for the past year. I had fitful sleeps, having already exhausted various investigations over the years looking for sleep apnea, trying and the weaning off sleeping pills after 2 years, and using bio-identical hormones to try to adjust for menopause (which at least got the hot flashes under control). My hands and feet were usually freezing or burning hot. I had mysterious choking episodes and swallowing issues so many times, that I was afraid I would actually choke and die every time. I had episodes of debilitating electric-shock-like tailbone pain and spasms that left me incapacitated, rocking and moaning on the floor, and these had been going on for over 8 years. Weird muscle twitches would happen anywhere in my body and at anytime, for no apparent reason. My mood swings were challenging and embarrassing to live with for me, let alone for Jeff! I could swing between anger, desperation, grief, sadness, irritability, restlessness, and impatience at a moment's notice. It was like constant PMS on steroids. Then I would just go emotionally numb.

Every day, I would get up, shower, get dressed, make a healthy breakfast — and do my best to hope today would be better. I could usually push myself to function through the first part of the day, but once I started to wane further, it was like falling off a cliff. Nothing was there...totally depleted. I had to lie down for a good part of the afternoon in order to make it through dinnertime. I would just about crawl up the stairs to bed early, night after night, in total despair.

Sometimes, even the effort of holding myself up in a chair to have a conversation would just be impossible. I had nothing left in me to be civil to anyone, or to physically manage anything, at those times. When a family member was frustrated with me for declining her invitation to a gathering, she barked at me: "All you have to do is just show up and sit there!" But often, I couldn't find one more ounce of will in myself to show up, and I couldn't sit there and listen or have a conversation. When I tried at that moment to tell her that I was having health issues that she wasn't aware of, and tears of frustration and hurt rolled down my face, she just angrily looked away and changed the subject.

With all this feedback, even from loved ones, I kept thinking I must be nuts. I felt ashamed and alone. Jeff and a couple of very close friends were really the only people who knew the extent of my symptoms and ongoing functional challenges. What kind of person gets these weird things that come and go? It didn't make sense, so I just stopped talking about it. I pretended to the outside world that I was just tired. I went mentally numb a lot, just to cope.

I distracted myself with reading and learning as much as I could, and trying to keep up at home with the household routines. I was grateful that my cognitive issues were not constant, and that I was so well-trained in health care that skimming medical articles online was enjoyable and doable for me for reasonable periods of time on some days. This also perplexed, me, though: if I could sit quietly at the computer at times and read articles, what was wrong with me at other times that I could hardly sit up to talk to anyone? The inconsistency of my ability further contributed to my embarrassment and shame.

Jeff's retirement

Remember that story from earlier — because of Jeff's work hours and my treatment schedule, it had taken months to have any decent time alone together. There was little time to reflect on the chaotic and unsustainable pace our lives had taken. This is the rest of the story of that day that Jeff and I were out for our drive.

As we were talking, something just snapped in me. This lifestyle, the insane one that we were trying to survive our way through, was wearing us both down. I just couldn't stand to go on like this any longer. We had to come up with something. Jeff looked constantly exhausted, and I didn't feel we could maintain this degree of stress without another health crisis occurring in one — *or both* — of us. Now that was a scary prospect, for sure.

"What would happen if you just put in your retirement notice now?" I asked out of the blue. "How long would it take before you could retire?" There was silence. He calculated. He was 58 and had been eligible to retire for a few years, but had kept working due to our extensive health care bills. "Around the beginning of August", he replied. That was just 3 months away. We just looked at each other and we knew we had to make it happen somehow.

Jeff retired on August 1, 2014. We celebrated that day by going over to our dear friend Lynda's for a quiet dinner for about two hours, and then I crashed again for the day. I had even spent the afternoon preparing for going out by doing extra resting and napping.

Having no real plan other than a good pension that we were very grateful for, and a few years of retirement savings that were rapidly dwindling due to my health care costs, we were alternately relieved and terrified about what might lie ahead for us financially. This was not how we planned to retire. In 2007, we had been two of many others who discovered we had lost our whole retirement savings, which was expected to amount to almost a million dollars by retirement, by investing in what turned out to be a criminal Ponzi scheme. We had two old vehicles that seemed to need frequent, expensive repairs. We still had a mortgage. But the present overwork situation had become intolerable, and Jeff's pension was similar to what he would make if he continued to work with no overtime.

Into Fall 2014: Taking charge in a new way

By the fall of 2014, Jeff and I were totally relieved by his retirement. The pressures of keeping up with daily life eased off significantly for me while having him home.

My energy was still very limited, but I began attacking my own health challenges in the way I have always approached my clients' issues. I had a strong determination to serve, to wonder, to ask and find out as much as possible, and to explore new options in order to solve the problem. I challenged my own beliefs and attitudes, and noticed where I was afraid of changing health professionals or courses of treatment and continually asked myself why.

I took charge at my appointments. I requested reviews of my case with each professional I was seeing, I quizzed them and pushed them to seek more insight. Based on their response or what they could or couldn't further offer me, I politely phased back or fired some of those practitioners and hired a few new ones.

I became more discerning and adept at hiring new professionals, not only with detailed questions asked to office staff but making direct email contact to see if they seemed to have the range of skills and curious attitude that I needed. After allowing what I thought was a reasonable time frame for getting some specific results, and based on an informed discussion with that professional, if their approach was not working I moved on to someone new. I watched to see who was really thinking about me and willing to explore new ideas, and who was just getting through my appointment, applying their tools as usual but lacking what I would later call "the wonder quotient" that was my new standard for my own care.

I searched website directories for lists of available local professional resources or those who would engage via Skype or a phone appointment but were outside of my area — in fact, I had to go outside of Canada to find the specialized resources I needed. I looked at 'who's who' in various functional medicine approaches and got to know who the key players were, and what their clinical approaches and treatment platforms seemed to be. I studied the online, international holistic health care industry. I listened to blog talk radio shows, and I asked questions on call-in shows to determine how those professionals would approach a complex, chronic case like mine.

I hit gold.

Once I got really good at finding expert, specific help, and checking it out more quickly and effectively, I booked a two-hour initial phone assessment with a USA-based practitioner. During the blur of busy months after that appointment, I did some more targeted lab testing in Canada and the USA, attended a few more trouble-shooting phone appointments, re-evaluated my diet, strategically adjusted my existing supplement program as recommended, and followed up on a medical referral.

Into 2015

Four months from that crucial new assessment, in March of 2015, Jeff and I emerged from a three-hour, in-person appointment in a Lyme Literate doctor's office with a clinical diagnosis of Lyme disease and possibly several co-infections. It had involved several days of travel by car and plane to the USA from Canada to get to this office, as well as considerable expense just for the expertise and consultation fees, but it was well worth every effort and every cent to us.

It had taken over 30 years to get here.

I was elated that I finally had a real diagnosis. Now the work of recovery from a real illness was beginning. Upon further specific lab testing in the ensuing weeks, along with clinical deliberation from my specialist, we finally knew what we were dealing with: chronic Lyme disease, Bartonella (a tick-borne co-infection), Chlamydia pneumonia (another nasty, complex bacterium that likely began with a respiratory infection, possibly as far back as high school), acute Epstein Barr virus, and acute Cytomegalovirus. It was a challenging, yet typical, 'Lyme cocktail' of pathogens. I had a pile of physical, mental and emotional symptoms, at times debilitating ones. I still had adrenal fatigue, hypothyroidism, and hormonal issues. I still had Chronic Fatigue Syndrome and Fibromyalgia, but now we knew much more about their underlying, associated — and treatable — pathogens. I had either gluten sensitivity or full-blown celiac disease (I had gone off gluten for a few years, and so did not undergo a definitive small intestine biopsy, but my genetic testing and clinical picture indicated this strong likelihood). I still had heavy metal toxicity and petrochemical toxicity. I was still actively dealing with various elements of emotional trauma, stemming from childhood and also from dealing with so many layers of grief and loss from chronic illness.

But even with all of this, the effect that having a 'real label' and a 'real reason' for all of this mess was freeing beyond what I had ever envisioned. I no longer felt I had to pretend to be well when I could hardly get through a day. We finally had names and a focus for what was going on, and with that insight, we could choose the best course of action. What I had was not easy to treat, but it was treatable.

I realized how much I had been blaming myself for something I could not overcome, despite all the years of holistic efforts and treatments I had consistently undergone. As I began to read and study voraciously about chronic Lyme disease, and about all of the issues with its diagnosis and treatment, I realized that my story was all too common: many years of mistaken reasons for illness, mysterious symptoms waxing and waning, and deep physical, emotional, mental and financial suffering. As relieved as I was, I also was terrified at what lay ahead of me with starting my chronic Lyme treatment.

My Pivotal Point in March 2015, And Turning 60

My journey was far from over. I had crossed a huge threshold, only to find that there were more challenges ahead. The first and immediate challenge was that my USA-based Lyme Literate Medical Doctor (LLMD) wanted me to start on three different antibiotics for treatment. Seems straightforward, right?

Well, not for me. I was forced to re-examine my own strong beliefs, once again. I had been Ms. Natural Treatments for most of my adult life. I couldn't stand the thought of undoing, with what I considered to be an 'evil' in antibiotics, all the hard work I had done in building up my system. For so many years, I had embraced the philosophy and practice that those natural remedies and methods were king. The thought of taking three new antibiotics paralyzed me so much that I felt I could literally not put them in my mouth. I was afraid I was going to go into anaphylaxis, die, or at least do irreparable harm to my liver and kidneys and gut.

How could I proceed with doing what I perceived to be poisoning myself with drugs? And how could I not? What were my options? Well, the long answer to this is content for bonus chapters — or another book!

First things first.

The short answer, that I believe will help you right now in your current path to *getting a diagnosis*, is that there are always more things that you can do — and need to do — in your Lyme diagnostic path and initial venture into recovery, instead of passively following the *physical remedy* treatment plan you are given. There is more to fully recovering from Lyme than just killing 'bugs' by your method of choice. The months of changing my habits and achieving actual progress after a long struggle is largely what gave rise to the guidance I have developed for you in Chapters Three, Four and Five of this book.

I realized in this phase of my journey that *getting a proper diagnosis* for a chronic, complex illness like Lyme disease requires some of the same tools, learned skills and processes that *recovering* from one does. In order to get my diagnosis, and set myself up for good recovery, I had to develop and apply my learned skills — most especially the following three skills:

1. **Navigating the medical system** and discerning all of the vast information and resources that could help me. **I had to learn how to be my own advocate**. I talk about how to develop and apply this skill in Chapter Three.

2. **Developing self-empowerment through strategic choices**. I had to learn how to **maximize my daily function**, to not only, in practical terms, better physically endure the whole long process of getting my diagnosis in the first place, but also to pace my way through the next phase of my life: starting Lyme treatment. This involved a lot of small but cumulative moment-by-moment choices that added up to me truly taking charge of my life. I learned that these choices really mattered. In Chapter Four, I discuss how self-empowerment can

be strengthened through the choices you make and where you place your day-to-day focus.

3. **Acknowledging mind, body and spirit connections. I learned that I had to build greater self-awareness to facilitate my recovery.** I had to understand how each of these aspects of myself directly and strongly affected the function of the other aspects. This growing awareness determined how I managed the complex medical aspects of my situation; how I lived and coped with limitations while I went through the long process of getting diagnosed; and how I would find my way through my recovery process. In Chapter Five, I take you beyond the common Lyme focus of external 'bug killing' treatment to introduce various internally-generated considerations and strategies for healing. Learning more about how your own system works, and how you can positively affect it, can set you up for successful recovery.

"How you do anything is how you do everything."
— *Ancient Proverb*

Back to my story of being on the threshold of finally initiating targeted Lyme treatment. Here was my unexpected complication: I was terrified, and soon realized I needed more tools to help me deal with even this, the severe anxiety that I had quietly carried within me for so many years. On the brink of finally having a solution, my anxiety was now getting in the way of being able to embark on the very treatment I needed, in order to help the thing I had been trying to identify for over 30 years. How totally ironic.

I knew somehow that my ongoing anxiety was physiological. It couldn't be separated out as being 'just' emotional or mental. I discovered, as I read further, that my anxiety was there for many reasons. It was due in part to Lyme and other co-pathogens affecting my brain and biochemistry. And it was also due to my history of emotional trauma, including many triggering life events, which had affected my nervous system. This knowledge led me to further important discoveries about the significant influence of past trauma in chronic illness, and the necessity for nervous system regulation. I learned that these are key influences upon creating a healing path for chronic Lyme disease.

I realized that I also needed to address the effects of these cumulative sources of stress and anxiety enough to judiciously plan and pursue some key treatment decisions. I needed to learn how I could possibly reduce many of the Lyme and co-infection symptoms that are usually attributed to 'just' pathogens. I'll describe more insight from this part of my journey in Chapter Five.

Chapter 3: Navigating the Medical System
Skill # 1: Be Your Own Advocate

"All advice is autobiographical…when people give you advice, they're really just talking to themselves in the past."
— *Austin Kleon, Steal Like an Artist* [60]

"When you have exhausted all possibilities, remember this: you haven't."
— *Thomas Edison*

By now you've learned about some of the very real challenges in trying to figure out what is going on with your health when you have symptoms across body systems, leading you to investigate a possible Lyme diagnosis. And you realize that even the process of getting that diagnosis is likely not going to be a straightforward matter of going to your family doctor, having a test done, a definitive diagnosis made, and starting treatment.

So now what? Where do you start on this diagnostic journey? How do you figure out the steps to take day by day, week by week?

The first step is a mindset step. You need to decide:

- That *you matter.*

- That *your health matters.*

- That *you have the right to full, expert medical investigation* about what is really going on.

- That you are willing to do *whatever it takes* to help yourself.

This is a decision that only you can make for yourself and your health. Yes, you'll need support. Yes, you'll need information. Yes, you'll need to build skills to help yourself in moving ahead. *But only you can decide that you're worth what it takes to walk this rocky road back to health.*

It doesn't matter what brings you to this place of determined grit. You can be angry, sad, fed up, lonely with your illness-imposed isolation, tired of feeling so sick for so long, tired of pretending, tired of trying to live up to the image of the life you were 'supposed' to have. *You will have to look the life you do have squarely in the eyes.*

That final event, or maybe the feeling state, that brings someone to this place of determined resolve is different for every one of us. It's that point where you know *that this is it.* But in order to find the strength and tenacity to move forward, you will have to find that place deep inside you that is now ready to draw a line in the sand and say, *"No more."*

Once you've reached that point, there are skills that you can learn and actions that you can take to move yourself forward. You will find that as you begin to make progress towards getting out of the vaguely understood, illness-dominated mess that you're in, life feels a whole lot better. It looks insurmountable from the bottom, and so you may have to trust that in making even a little bit of progress and viewing your life from different vantage point, life will become substantially better.

Your Role as General Contractor of your Health

What does it mean to fully take charge of your health? For most of us, this is new territory. It is important to *learn how to be proficient* in this new terrain in order to be able to function in a demanding new way to achieve what you want: a diagnosis.

Being assertive with your own health care needs and goals isn't something you'll just innately know how to do. That's why I describe it as a *learned skill*. Most of us are not taught this in our youth. Believe me, it was a concept that just slowly began to dawn upon me as I realized I still had a lot to learn to get through my own process. I got better at it with a lot of frustrating, inefficient, and expensive trial and error over many years.

The skills you'll need in order to become your own medical investigator and health advocate are ones that tend to develop from desire to find answers, awareness of what you do and don't know, and practice. This pretty much applies to any new thing you've learned in life, and since you've been alive for a likely a few decades or more, you already have that going for you. So perhaps you aren't learning fundamental skills here, but refining a new practical, specialized application for them.

In this Lyme investigation world, and perhaps anywhere in the world of chronic illness, you can no longer be a passive patient. Regardless of how scared, helpless, overwhelmed, angry or foggy you feel, you'll need to take full responsibility for your own health care at each step of the way. There will be days that you feel too sick to bother or too foggy or overwhelmed to proceed. That will happen, so don't beat yourself up for it. Just get back to it as soon as you can and don't give up.

There is a phrase that's been developed in recent years for people who are powerfully taking charge of their health care. They see themselves as working in equal partnership with their health care providers, and use extensive online resources in order to seek out key medical information and make complex health care decisions. These people are called *e-patients*.[61]

Dave deBronkart, known as "e-patient Dave", delivered a very powerful TED talk[62] about his positive health outcome in beating a rare and usually terminal cancer in 2007, thanks to his self-advocacy work as an e-patient. He continues to advocate for widely opening health care information to patients in order to create a stronger patient-doctor dialogue, better access to information, and more favorable health outcomes.

Dave deBronkart has also commented that patient empowerment and advocacy is actually now becoming a civil rights movement.[63]

Being your own strong, informed advocate doesn't mean that you can't or shouldn't defer to medical judgments or professional recommendations. But it does mean that you'll need to view the personnel that you consult about your health as just that: *consultants*. Whether medical, allied or holistic health, specialist or generalist, you can choose to see them all as consultants, rather than absolute authorities. They are human beings with skills and flaws. They are personnel that you are hiring to help you get a job done: the job of finding out what is wrong with you, so you can do something about it.

This will help you keep the attitude that you are the one in charge here, so that you can abide in your own quiet power and get your questions answered. This will be necessary in order to get the help you need. It does not have to mean being harsh, abrasive, rude or ungrateful. But it does mean that you have to give up the illusion that all medical personnel have all the answers, or even that they always ask all the relevant questions. They don't. And medical diagnostic and treatment answers are often not the clear black-and-white realities that we've been led to believe. That's why medicine is also an art, not just a science. But the right health care resource people often will have more answers than you do, and you need them in your corner. Making the most of your whole diagnostic experience so that you can get the clarity you need is critical.

Even though I have many years of experience being on both sides of the diagnostic desk and treatment table as a health professional and as a patient, I am still learning this valuable lesson. There have been so many frustrating medical appointments in my own background — ones where I have left angry, sometimes insulted, dismissed or badly treated. I questioned the usefulness of the appointment, doubted myself, and felt like I was no further ahead. And there have been times that I was so grateful for the compassionate help I received that I just wanted to hug the doctor (and sometimes did!).

When I realized that the outcome of any given appointment was drastically affected by my own action — how I prepared for it (or didn't), the attitude and expectations I went in with, and how I conducted myself and presented my own medical information in the appointment — everything changed for me. I finally felt in charge and in my own power, while at the same time being an eager consumer of the (often excellent) services provided for me.

Health care professionals, your consultants, function in all kinds of ways. Some are personable and service-oriented, and some are crabby. Some are fully present with you and determined to help with all the amazing tools and brainpower they can muster, and some see you as the next case on their list to get through as fast as possible — maybe because they are already stressed and behind in their day and you are keeping them from finally having their much-needed break for lunch. The sooner you can take them off a pedestal and just see them as highly trained people with awesome, yet finite skills that may either help you tremendously, may not help you at all, or even make you worse — the better equipped you are to navigate the health care system full of human beings.

Skill building 101: Navigating your health care appointments

There are some key lessons that I learned by trial and error. I hope that by providing you with these tips, your expectations may be considered — making the whole medical investigation process a smoother and less emotionally harrowing one for you.

You'll need to fully prepare for each health care appointment. This includes the following measures:

1.   Knowing why you are going for the consultation, what that specialty's expertise is and isn't, and anything you specifically need to bring or do ahead of time.

Knowing all of this ahead of time will save you a lot of frustration, and will help you to be realistic about what can and can't happen in a given appointment. You may want to look up an unfamiliar medical specialty online during your preparation, and see what their scope of practice is, the kinds of things they test for, and how those tests may be experienced.

Call and find out from the office staff how long the appointment booking is for. If it is for assessment only, ask if there will also be any testing done that day, or will another day be required. Is there anything that could be ordered and completed ahead of time? If it is an in-person appointment, do you need to go early to fill out forms? How lengthy are the intake forms? Could they be emailed or mailed to you a few days prior so that you can do them on a day when your energy is higher, and either send them ahead or bring them with you? This will help you plan your time, energy and expectations for the service that's being provided, as well as anticipate and accommodate logistics such as your transportation and meals.

Understanding the skills and limitations of that medical specialty's role as well as being aware of your own expectations and needs, can really affect the outcome of your consultation experience.

For example, at a conventional cardiology initial consultation I attended, my rational mind knew that the symptoms that the physician was interested in assessing would be ones pertaining to my heart and circulation only. Yet somehow, my desperation for new health care answers outweighed that factual knowledge. I went into that consultation unaware of my own considerable neediness for those answers. After we reviewed the findings of the previous cardiac tests I had completed, he told me my heart appeared to be fine. I then found myself desperately gushing forth with my huge list of symptoms, hoping in vain that someone would take me seriously. Responding to my desperate tone, he rapidly stood up and nudged me out the door, and asked me on the way out, "Have you considered that anxiety could be the cause of all your symptoms?" In frustration, I told him that the anxiety I felt about my health seemed to be the result of having so many symptoms for so many years with no answers. I went home feeling horribly frustrated and misunderstood yet again, but I also knew it was my own conduct that added to the negative experience.

My Lesson learned: recognize the parameters of the given specialty, and contain your comments and questions only to that area. Regard it as the useful insurance-covered screening that it is: finding or ruling out any overt pathology in that one field of medicine. Don't try bringing brain, nervous system and emotion-related symptoms — like severe fatigue, brain fog, vertigo, muscle twitching or concentration issues — to a cardiologist, just because you are finally so glad to see someone who spends time with you and treats you well. Your secret hope your symptoms may be seen as real, and may even be heart-related in some way, is only your attachment to your outcome at work here. Know the predisposition of your own mind, and be prepared to keep things in check as required.

2. Bring your own well-organized medical reports to each appointment. As the person who is fully in charge of your whole health care picture, you'll need to get a copy of everything medical you've done in the past few years (and any key reports from even longer back historically) and put it in a three-ring binder.

Ask each medical office you attend to mail or fax you a copy of all tests and reports, and follow up if they forget. This is your legal right. Don't expect that it will be done for you without asking, or that they will arrive on time to the next referral without verifying that they were sent and received. Call ahead of each appointment and be sure all necessary reports are there before you go, if something has been forwarded from another doctor or lab.

If you can afford to buy a fax machine to use for receiving and sending pages of medical reports, I have found that it is a real time and energy saver. You can set it up on your existing phone line with a distinctive ring, so that you don't have to pay for a separate phone line. You can also install a fax app or use an online service that sends and receives faxes. Otherwise, many reports can now be scanned on a printer/scanner and sent by email. You may find that you need to do a combination of both and also snail mail, depending on the state of electronic set-up or preferences in any particular medical office.

Separate your conventional health care records from any complementary or alternative health care records, tests and reports, with labeled dividers in your binder. That way each specialty can easily access just what they need or wish to review during your appointment. My Lyme physician was overstressed, overscheduled and subsequently irate with me at our initial consultation. Because I had followed her office staff's general directions to "bring everything that you have with you," I handed her a huge pile of tests, many of which were my complementary health professionals' lab testing. It turned out she wanted *conventional medical reports only*, and those to be presented in chronological order. My pile of reports, and painstakingly grouped re-tests of the same type, overwhelmed her and sent her off track for the time we had available, especially given my long and complex history. It turned out a poor use of her time as well as mine.

Have a full medical history prepared, chronologically from birth until present, on a typed document that you keep on your computer and update that regularly. Include significant life events that were stressful or disruptive, too — ones such as family deaths, financial, work or marital status changes. Include a present list of all of your symptoms, and a separate document of all supplements and drugs, including over the counter preparations, you are taking either regularly or occasionally. This may take you a few weeks of preparation, as you may find yourself needing to go back and add to it as you remember various details. Include this in your binder and bring it with you to all new appointments. It will save you a lot of unnecessary energy output by having it all organized in one place. It also will be a big help to your health professionals, in being able to copy whatever information they need in order to help their own diagnostic workup.

3.   Prepare a written list of prioritized questions and bring them to each appointment. Designate a file folder for each medical consultant, and a keep files organized in a system at home. Some people prefer crates or tabletop files, others invest in a secure cabinet for this purpose, depending on the volume of paperwork you must manage. Still others rely on saving records electronically. Keep your questions together with the date of each appointment and notes from any previous appointments. Organize your questions in strict numbered priority, *starting with what you can't stand to leave the phone or in-person appointment without knowing.* Find out how much time you have at the beginning of your appointment, and use your time wisely. Stick to the brief facts as you ask or answer questions, and keep your feelings under wraps to be handled by another professional whose specialty it is to help you with emotional support. The more you can stick to objective facts and concisely report those to the professional, the more they can have a clear head to problem solve your situation.

Utilizing Your Family Physician as a Home Base of Support

Your family physician's role, and your relationship with him or her, may change anywhere from mildly to drastically when you're dealing with a decision to undergo further investigation of your suspicion that you may have chronic Lyme disease. The family physician's role may tend to vary from one physician to another, based on their location and scope of practice, insurance regulations, their own office structure and particular areas of interest and expertise.

In my own case, my family physician of over 25 years does five-minute appointments, and has a very efficient office structure, so I rarely wait very long. He is very polite and supportive in making referrals that I inquire about or request, to the various insurance-covered medical specialty professionals in our immediate geographic area. For example, if it's determined by my symptoms that I may need a conventional cardiologist, neurologist, or endocrinologist to assess me to check for any pathology, then he is an excellent resource. If I have concerns that may require insurance-covered blood testing or other screening tests, it's done quickly from his requisition slip given to me. If I need a routine physical, I can book one, and he will check the usual vital information, such as my heart rate, blood pressure, routine blood work, or administer a pap test.

This is all fine to help with an acute situation that may require an examination or meds (eg. antibiotics for acute bronchitis) or routine Western medical, insurance-covered screening (eg. a colonoscopy requisition). As long as my complaint is clear, is something that Western medicine can handle, and takes less than 5 minutes to discuss and to leave with the relevant referral slip or prescription, it's all fine. And it's much appreciated for the easy access, the mutual respect, and longevity of the professional relationship.

Where it totally falls apart is that it is not realistic to

fully assess or treat complex, chronic disease or illness in the primary care office. This cannot be done in 5 minutes, nor is it the family physician's role to even try to figure this out. It is beyond their scope of practice, insured time frame, expertise or inclination. *Our system is just not set up for this.*

So if you've only accessed the whole medical world through this family physician's door, what do you do now? You've maxed out his or her expertise and time, as well as that of the various insured specialty physicians they have sent you to. You may or may not have acquired several labels by now, all of which are accurate from the best expertise of the specialty that assessed you and the insured tests that they are approved to use. You may have been told you are "fine," that there is nothing showing up that is beyond the normal parameters of usual testing, or that they just don't know what is wrong.

Although you may have seen a lot of proficient doctors by now, *Lyme was never on anyone's radar at all.*

You may be disheartened, feel like you're crazy, and may be on meds that do or don't have any positive effect, in an attempt to relieve various symptoms. You're still not satisfied. Your intuition tells you that you can do better; that there is really something going on that just has not been found. You feel it, you know it, and you are not ready to give up on yourself and stop investigating.

You've made a big decision: It's time to look elsewhere.

Before you jump ship completely in frustration, and dismiss your family doctor as no help, please keep in mind that he or she can still help you — and his role is still very valuable. As you continue your search elsewhere, keep going back, and keep them informed. Keep an open dialogue going. Discuss together how they can help you in a slightly different role: that of continuing with support of insured services to supplement the work that you are doing with other professionals that are 'outside the system'. He has to work within the system that governs his legal practice, his health insurance payments, and his livelihood. *But that doesn't mean that you have to stay totally within those boundaries.*

I have been very grateful to my family doctor, who has continued to support me over the years within his role limitations, by giving me access to insured services when I need them. This has saved me a lot of time, money, and aggravation, and more importantly has continued to allow me continuity of acute care and access to conventional health screening as needed. I just learned to recognize that his role has considerable limitations for someone like me with a complex chronic illness. *It is a systems issue. It's not personal.*

Finding your own 'Generalist Specialist' and Lyme Literate Medical Help

I first heard the term *'generalist specialist'* from my USA-based current health care 'detective/practitioner' Shawn Bean and his business partner, Dr. Jess Armine.[64] It was Shawn Bean who led me to my Lyme Literate physician. Jess and Shawn have coined this term to describe the lost art and science of applying a discerning, logical, holistic problem-solving view to the client when assessing their health situation.

Assessment needs to include current symptoms, key lab findings and extensive history when evaluating a complex chronic illness. This process takes considerable time spent with the client, and broad general knowledge combined with specific expertise and experience. It also requires what I have come to call *"The Wonder Quotient"*.

I have come to learn that some professionals have this *Wonder Quotient* and some just don't. Or maybe they had it at one time, but now they're so overwhelmed or burned out from years of service that they can't muster it anymore. It's the one quality that now determines a make-or-break hiring or firing of professionals for me, when I need health care help.

What is the *Wonder Quotient?* This key quality is what drives professionals to excellence. They just can't stop thinking, wondering, learning and discovering. They are rabid consumers of health information in their field. Give them a complicated case, and they like to think about it even on their time off. This is *fun* for them! They love taking on cases that others have not been able to solve. Their egos are firmly parked at the door, because they know that what they know already (which is very extensive in most of these cases) is always just the tip of the iceberg. They know that their learning will never stop. They also let their clients teach them. Their curiosity is unparalleled. They are primo detectives in the health care world.

Who would you rather have working on your case, one that you may have spent years trying to solve, but still to no avail? Do you want an enthusiastic health detective with a *Wonder Quotient?* Or someone who tends to be satisfied with the status quo in their field, and for whatever extensive practical or temperamental reasons, puts in solid days on the job, yet has no burning curiosity to solve complex health riddles like yours?

So how do you find these health care detectives who possess the *Wonder Quotient?* By being a health care detective *yourself!*

Using the Internet to help you

The internet has changed the face of health care. You now have access to anything you want to know about. That is good news and bad news. Especially if this kind of exploration is new to you, it can be overwhelming to know where to start, and how to determine whether what you've found is going to be of any use to you or not.

Here are some questions that you may have about how to proceed with online investigations and how to find resources to help you in your quest. These are focused on finding the right person to assess you for Lyme, and include some additional suggestions that you may want to try.

Q: What kind of 'generalist specialist' or 'health care detective' do I look for? What are their areas of expertise and training?

A: You may find that these people come from a variety of original professional backgrounds, and then have undergone further professional training that has led them away from the way their profession is usually practiced. Their original professional training may include diverse fields such as nutrition, chiropractic, homeopathy, naturopathy, Chinese medicine, or various fields within conventional medicine. Their subsequent health care training and experience will also vary, but will tend to be focused holistically from the standpoint that they do long and detailed client assessments, and will set out to look for the root cause(s) of your illness. The clue you are looking for in reading descriptions about what these people do is that in assessing you, *they are looking to identify some kind of (as yet unidentified) pathogenic activity or inflammatory process that is likely at the root of your chronic illness.* And they are set up to evaluate your system as a whole, including your history, symptoms, immune system status, nutritional status, genetic influences, function of biochemical pathways and other details. If you search terms like "diagnosis of Lyme disease," or "assessing chronic illness", as well as "holistic approach" alongside diagnoses like fibromyalgia, chronic fatigue syndrome, MS, and autoimmune diseases, you will find a wide range of resources. You can also look for categories of practitioners that aim to assess and treat root cause of illness, like bio-individualized medicine, functional medicine or integrated medicine.

A good practitioner who is Lyme aware and excellent at evaluating chronic illness, but who does not necessarily fully treat Lyme, can be an invaluable resource in screening you to start you on your Lyme diagnostic path. They can also recommend how you can optimize your health while awaiting your specific Lyme referral and workup, and may continue to work with you for holistic support while you undergo Lyme treatment. They are able to fill in the treatment areas such as health-boosting nutritional and supplement support, that are outside the scope of a Lyme

MD's practice. I'll expand more of this later on building your health care team.

Q: What kind of titles do they have that are searchable online?

A: They may go by their original training's degree or title (eg. MS in Nutrition, DC, MD, ND, D Hom, D.C.M., D.O.M., etc.), or they may have a title such as a Doctor of Functional or Integrative Medicine. They may describe that they evaluate people with various chronic illnesses or syndromes such as fibromyalgia or chronic fatigue syndrome. They may list that they specialize in treating Lyme disease. Some well-known Lyme specialists do not have a website, and may be only accessed by word of mouth or referrals whether by other patients, former patients, or health care providers.

Q: How do I know if what I have going on health-wise is legitimately suspicious of Lyme 'enough' to warrant seeing a Lyme specialist?

A: If you think you may have Lyme, you deserve to have this checked out by a competent health care professional who is current with leading practices in Lyme testing and clinical evaluation. You will have to contact the Lyme specialist's office or look at their website, if they have one, to see what their criteria are for accepting new patients for evaluation.

There are some Lyme specialists, including some who you can find through Lyme online searches who will do a Skype or phone consultation with you at a reasonable cost to help you determine if your symptoms warrant a full medical assessment. Don't let the fear or possible embarrassment of not being 'sick enough' or having 'enough' Lyme symptoms stop you from inquiring. If you do a preliminary phone consultation to inquire further about evaluating for Lyme, be sure to have all of your medical materials and history with you as outlined earlier. This time it is primarily a tool for yourself, so that you have everything you need at your fingertips to discuss during a brief consultation with a new person.

Q: Should I see a Lyme specialist right away, or should I look for some other kind of person that will then refer me to the 'Lyme Literate' specialist, LLMD or LLND?

A: You could do either. Be aware that each health care professional will have their specific areas of clinical expertise as well as their limitations and biases.

Although there is less variation in how the LLMD or LLND will lab test and clinically assess you to diagnose Lyme and co-infections, there is a wide range of ways in which they treat it. The Lyme MD or ND may or may not use any number of conventional or holistic approaches in their treatment.

This is where it can get tricky. At this point, you are looking to just see if you have Lyme and/or co-infections, and to get a diagnosis once and for all. However, if you are satisfied with the LLMD or LLND who assesses you, likely you will want to continue with them to supervise your treatment program. If so, you may wish to read a bit about the various approaches to treatment for Lyme & co-infections, to see what an individual LLMD or LLND offers.

There are many, many books and blogs written about the

challenges and controversies associated with chronic Lyme and co-infection treatment. There are conventional drugs, natural herbal and energy medicine approaches, and combinations of those. Right now, you want to get a diagnosis, but will need to have some awareness of treatment protocols so that you can factor your preferences or comforts in to the decision of where you will go for assessment.

Q: What about complimentary health professionals who specialize in Lyme disease? Am I limited only to medical doctors to help me?

A: Occasionally you will find a complimentary health care professional who is Lyme Literate and very experienced in using natural approaches for treating chronic Lyme and co-infections. Examples I have seen online are Doctors of Chinese Medicine and Acupuncture, Homeopathy and Naturopathy. You may decide to go directly with this option instead of accessing the expertise of a LLMD or LLND. You will need to screen them as well, and find out if they require a formal clinical and lab-tested diagnosis of Lyme from an LLMD or LLND before treating you, or if they will perform diagnostics.

Varying levels of expertise in Lyme disease diagnosis also exists among 'on the grid' mainstream medical specialists and complimentary health care professionals. Just because someone is expertly trained in Western medicine or in natural medicine and has experience with chronic illness, does not mean they are also proficient in diagnosing Lyme disease. You will always need to do your own due diligence and determine the best-qualified professional for your needs.

Q: Most of the Lyme resources I've found online so far seem to be in the USA and I live in Canada. Can I find someone here, or do I have to travel to the USA to get help?

A: We have a problem with scarcity of Lyme resources here in Canada for diagnosis and treatment. Our insured testing and physician-approved diagnostic guidelines for Lyme disease, as mentioned in Chapter One, are very narrow — and in my opinion, inadequate. Continue to check the *Canadian Lyme Disease Foundation* website, www.canlyme.com for additional health care resources and recommendations. You may find that you likely need to go out of Canada to find the resources you need for clinical diagnosis and specialized laboratory testing, due to the limitations of what is done in our provincial laboratories.

You have the right to consult with anyone you wish. But you will have to find a way to pay for it, as the only financial recourse we have in Canada when exploring beyond local, insured resources is to submit your expenses for a bit of an income tax break on your health care costs. So keep all of your receipts, including travel for each appointment, if that is the diagnostic route you end up taking.

If you need to get a blood draw for a test that you've been told is only done in the USA, or you're not sure what is or is not covered by your provincial health care plan, you have a few options:

- First, be sure that your US-based LLMD has clearly named and described all requested tests and test panels on the requisition, as the names can vary from the US to Canada.

- You can look up the test names online, and see what is funded by your provincial health care plan. Print out the names of the funded tests.

- Speak to the manager of your local blood draw laboratory about the specific tests required, and clarify what can and cannot be done locally, and what is and isn't covered by your provincial insurance. You may be able to do some tests locally, but have to pay out of pocket for them because they are not standard, provincially-insured ones. If you have extended health care insurance coverage from an employer or your spouse's employer, check to see if any lab testing will be covered under that plan. This coverage will vary from one company to another.

- If a US-based lab is needed for some tests that your LLMD or LLND requires, because they are not offered at all here in Canada, you will need to arrange access to a US lab.

- If you live close to a US border, you can drive to a US lab for on-site testing. Otherwise, you may be able to co-ordinate the proper preparation and sending of blood samples to a US lab from your local lab. You will need to pay shipping expenses and lab fees out of pocket and co-ordinate the details of this yourself as your case is now sole responsibility for neither your local lab, nor the US lab.

You may also need to order supplements and drugs from the USA, if you do have Lyme and co-infections, and you do pursue treatment from a US-based practitioner. I want to reassure you that all of this is possible to co-ordinate, and you can find a way to sort out all of the necessary details. You may find that your US-based practitioner has some experience with Canadian patients, or that your Canadian friends have experience with US-based practitioners. Although it can be time-consuming and there may be a lot of red tape, when you want to get help with these aspects of diagnosis and treatment, I believe that avenue is well worth pursuing.

Some of the things that you may want to look for in your search and consider before hiring a LLMD or LLND are:

- Does this professional assess and treat only in person, or also by Skype and phone (or a combination of contacts)?

- Where are they located in relation to you, and how does the above information affect your hiring decision?

- How do they accept referrals? Is it through other doctors or health professionals only, or also available by direct patient request?

- What are their consultation fees?

- How long are the assessment and follow-up appointments, and what is the frequency of follow-up?

- How long does it take to get an initial appointment?

- What is their process for evaluation, including types and costs of usual lab testing required and recommended?

- What methods do they use (or not use) for treatment, and how does that fit with your preferred approach?

- Are they affiliated with any other professionals that work with them as a complimentary team member to co-ordinate with other aspects of your care? (eg. nutritionist, Naturopath)

- How long has it already been that you have been looking for answers? Do you want to hold out for the perfect scenario, or go to a good resource that you can get into ASAP, and decide later what you will do about treatment options, if you do indeed have Lyme? This can be a viable question to consider also.

Q: What's the difference between LLMD and LLND anyway?

A: It depends on where they practice, which affects their scope of practice. This determines the medical testing they can and can't do by law, and influences the selection of conventional and holistic or natural treatments that they provide. You will need to inquire individually. LLMD is a Medical Doctor by training, and LLND is a doctor of Naturopathy.

Here are some further online search tips when looking for resources for your own 'health care detective' or Lyme literate MD/ND:

- Functional or integrative medicine practitioners can be found by direct search, or by searching their professional organizations, which often contain practitioner listings by location.

- Facebook groups or forums, chat rooms on Lyme or other chronic illnesses that you have been labeled with already, can be found via a Facebook search or by using your general search engine. See who is talking about which practitioners, who they've had success with, and why they are satisfied or not.

- Amazon searches can yield general books on Lyme. Check out authors' names, then search them online for articles, practice locations, blogs, and other publications.

- Sign up for any free holistic health summits you can find that relate to Lyme diagnosis or to aspects of chronic illness often related or coinciding with Lyme such as: chronic fatigue syndrome, fibromyalgia, MS. See who the key players are, attend some of their online lectures, and search their websites.

- Read online articles & blog posts, and listen to podcasts or blog talk radio shows on Lyme and related topics in investigating chronic illness. See what you think of that person's area of expertise. Is it what you need?

- Ask your questions via blog talk radio shows, online forums, chat rooms, and direct email listed in the contact section of the practitioners' websites.

Tips for Making a decision about who to hire

Once you've narrowed down your search to a handful of professionals who appeal to you for various reasons, it's time to get more details about their practice. Here are some tips for making your final decision about whom to start with:

- *Set up your list of questions you'll need to find answers to.* These may include any of the above-mentioned questions for new practitioners or the ones that are unique to your personal priorities and health history. Get the answers you can online, and then call their office or email to get the rest. Keep all of this clearly organized in a new file folder with a separate page for each professional.

- *Decide on your budget.* This can be a harrowing experience, depending upon your own financial situation. For many of us, going down the Lyme diagnostic and treatment road, finding a means for more income has been a sobering requirement. This may involve temporary use of credit cards, new mortgages or bank loan financing, using savings (all of which we have done), borrowing from family or friends, or doing online or private fund raising. Don't let this hurdle stop you if you can at all find some creative means to finance your health needs. I know this is not pretty. You may need to investigate this online as well, to find out how others have obtained fund raising for their health journey.

- *Use your intuition or access some intuitive*

methods to help with decision-making.

Sometimes available health care access and associated costs will end up narrowing your decision down fairly quickly, using just your logical mind and a quick gut feel. Do your searching in small increments of time, and come back to it a few times, so you don't get too overwhelmed. Make decisions when you are able to think and feel clearly about what you need and what you want to do.

Trust that you will know what feels right for you. With your exploration, you'll develop a sense of what is out there, what suits you, and what doesn't. You'll feel attracted to or repelled by certain resources for various reasons. You'll need to honestly evaluate what you are willing and able to do physically, mentally and financially to access your chosen resources. Make it your intention that the right resources will show up to help you, and be aware of what appears, and what subtle clues may confirm your gut reactions. There are many methods that can be learned to help you make decisions related to your health care by directly accessing and building upon your own innate intuition.

There are also skilled, certified practitioners in the growing field of Medical Intuition who can access specific, helpful information about your mind, body and spirit. This information can be considered by you and your health care team when making decisions about what may need to be further investigated or treated, based on important physiological interconnections that may have eluded your awareness. For those who have no experience with this field, you may be skeptical (as I was, even while receiving my medical intuition certification training[65] — it was just all so new and I had a lot of societal conditioning to overcome to even consider it!). Learning more about quantum physics and energy fields helped me to understand the science behind how it is possible to access this rich, unseen yet very real source of information. If it interests you to explore this further, my mentor Lori Wilson's book, *Demystifying...Medical Intuition*[66] is a good place to start.

In my client coaching practice, I like to include accessing your own body-felt intuition as an area of skill building. I find it builds confidence and self-trust for all areas of life decisions. These intuition-building tools may include applied kinesiology (also called muscle testing) and various body awareness tools.

Building (and Re-building) your Health Care Team

You may have already pursued several rounds of specialists, and rounds of complementary health care treatments, like I did. You may be actively involved in ongoing treatment from one or several heath care professionals right now. You may be dealing with and treating any combination of adrenal fatigue, fibromyalgia, thyroid issues, food sensitivities, leaky gut, various toxic exposure issues, chronic fatigue syndrome or other diagnostic labels. That doesn't mean that those labels have gone away or that they just disappear when you get a Lyme diagnosis. They will still need to be dealt with. But what may be happening is that although you have those conditions, the underlying root or stress in your system may also include undiagnosed pathogens like Lyme and other co-infections or viruses. *If you have pursued and co-operated with long-term treatment and find you are still not well, I believe that it is worth it to have Lyme properly ruled in or out, in case it is a missing key to your health picture.* The "great imitator" called Lyme can fool so many competent health professionals and even highly-aware patients.

If you have a multi-symptom condition, then you've likely already accessed a significant number of professional resources. But if your health care experience to date has consisted mostly of working *within* the insured health care system, and especially through the filter of one primary health care professional like your family physician, the concept of building an ongoing health care 'team' may be a new one for you.

Building your own health care team is based upon the conscious implementation of the concept that each health care professional possesses an "information wall" which is a term I think is so aptly named, one that I first heard from Shawn Bean.[67] They have areas of expertise that are well-defined, based on their education, legislated scope of practice, and their own preferences and experience.

In Chapter One, I mentioned that one of the issues with chronic Lyme is that it has a multi-faceted cause —

i.e. in order for Lyme to have successfully outrun your own immune system's ability to fight it off, along with likely other co-infections, there has to be some kind of faltering within your immune system. Which pathogen or life stressor came first, and exactly how this vicious cycle continued to result in your perfect storm of ill health, can be tough to determine.

In order to manage for the long-term, starting *right now* as you are looking into getting a Lyme diagnosis, you are going to need to address your health from a multi-faceted perspective. Although the killing of 'bugs' is paramount, and may be a key addition to your current attempt to get well, the way in which that is done can vary greatly and is best overseen by an experienced LLMD or LLND.

Your own health care team will likely consist of professionals who come from a range of backgrounds. Just like you need to choose your key medical professional (e.g. your LLMD or LLND) to provide an overview and level of expertise, they cannot and will not have all of the health-enhancing tools you need. You will need to assess which pieces are missing from your care and consider how to best access the trained personnel to fill those gaps. These people may include a physiotherapist, a massage therapist, a nutritionist; a naturopathic, homeopathic or osteopathic doctor; a doctor of Chinese medicine and acupuncture; a counselor, life coach, therapist, body worker or energy worker such as a reflexologist; or many other types of professionals including your 'health care detective', coming from various backgrounds. You are treating body, mind, emotions, and spirit here, and your professionals should reflect that composite.

As general contractor for your health care, your job includes hiring and firing of your personnel. This means that you are always the one in charge, and you need to assess the qualifications, practice and effectiveness of anyone you hire. You need to maintain your own power, while you hire people as your consultants. This implies that you collaborate with them to set clear parameters about what they can and cannot do for you, what information they need to access and share with other team members, how you can co-operate fully to maximize their help, how their role fits into the rest of the team, and how information gets communicated between team members.

When their care — along with your considerable, co-operative efforts — is no longer meeting the expectations and guidelines that you have set up together, ones you mutually agreed to be reasonable and achievable in moving you to a better state of health, you fire (or simply replace) them and move on.

This job as general contractor for your own health starts *now*. It started the moment you drew that line in the sand and said, *"No more!"* You said *no* to being powerless, victimized or hopeless. You said *no* to waiting a moment longer in the state you're in, hoping that somehow this health mess will change on its own. *It hasn't.* So now it's up to you to make change happen.

Chapter 4: Self-Empowerment Through Strategic Choices
Skill # 2: Maximize Your Daily Function

"A hero is an ordinary individual who finds the strength to persevere and endure in spite of overwhelming obstacles."
— *Christopher Reeve* [68]

This journey towards a new diagnosis is a daunting task of its own. By the end, you will either get a Lyme and co-infection diagnosis or at least rule it out conclusively. When you've been sick for so long, and feel unsatisfied with the answers you've been given, wondering if you have Lyme is not just an academic question — it's a personal one. It's *your life and your whole future* we're talking about here!

Having a diagnosis of Lyme and several co-infections changed everything for me. It gave me the opportunity to drastically improve my quality of life by knowing and addressing what is really going on. Finally, I have a 'real thing' to target in my comprehensive approach *that is treatable*. No more vague concepts or guesswork. The far-reaching psychological effects for me, as a result of finally obtaining the Lyme diagnosis, have been significant. I was finally able to start moving past shame, guilt and self-recrimination which infiltrated my way of operating for most of my adult life. I had a reason for feeling so badly. I had a *real name* that I could give my family and friends to relate my suffering, instead of just another vague excuse for not attending something because I felt too ill or exhausted. Finally, I could make sense of over 30 years of my life. The relief related to simply knowing the 'culprit' has been incredible.

The diagnosis of Lyme disease and any associated co-infections can change how you feel about yourself by finally realizing your health issues are 'legitimate'. You're not crazy or imagining all of these strange symptoms after all. Diagnosis can give you a real entity to understand and to learn about, so that you can discover the various current approaches to treatment. It gives you a framework from which you can move forward to determine your best course of treatment and who you will choose to help guide you through it. It may even save your life, by treating something that is actually treatable, rather than letting it take its natural course by default as when the insight of this diagnosis is not available. If left untreated, the risk is that these pathogens will wreak havoc on your brain and nervous system. This means the disease will likely progress, the symptoms of which may be labeled as some other neurological disease such as ALS, for which there has been no known cure.[69]

As you are well-aware, there are a number of steps that you will need to follow, and factors to consider at each step, in order to get a Lyme diagnosis. There are decisions to be made and a lot of possible professional health care resources to evaluate and assess as potential partners. There are medical professionals' timetables and availability that will affect you also, but over which you have no control. This whole diagnostic process is likely *not* one that will happen overnight, and in fact it may take weeks or months yet.

On top of you *still being sick and fed up with still being sick*, and while trying to cope with all the demands of day-to-day life, you unfortunately have a whole new project: finding out if your actual diagnosis is Lyme or not. Before you throw this book down in full blown exasperation, fear and overwhelm, let's talk about how you can steadily prepare yourself for your new diagnostic journey ahead.

Likely your energy is significantly limited, along with having to manage a host of other symptoms. So that means that the idea of adding new, unfamiliar things to your already overfull to-do list does not really thrill you and may threaten to send you into hibernation, avoidance, or meltdown. I get it. I still feel that way on my worst days when I'm trying to make a new decision, hire a new professional, or re-evaluate the professional help that I have already hired.

I have to admit that managing my significant energy limitations has been a constant challenge for me. Some days, and some weeks, I do a better job of it than others. At other times, I realize too late that I've way over-extended myself due to taking care of what I thought I *really needed* to do, or doing what I *really wanted* to do. The results have been miserable days of worsening symptoms, cancellations of various commitments and entire life plans, and a forced ramping up of rest and recovery time.

So what are you to do? How in the world can you

navigate *your life* through a whole new set of activities that will involve personally taking on the flawed medical system, to find your way through unfamiliar territory, and deeper into further, as yet unknown, options?

What I introduce in this chapter is tools that will help you build your awareness and skills in dealing with key areas of day-to-day life, so that you can make the most of the function that you have. There are common struggles that people have in general with chronic illness that will continue to be a reality — or will be even more amplified — while you are undergoing more diagnostic investigation.

Taking control of your own daily life involves a constant series of decisions and steps. The decisions you make and steps you learn to take will either bring you closer to a feeling of self-empowerment or to a dismal state of passivity and victimhood. How you live your life and take charge of it is that important. And it is up to you.

In this chapter I help you craft your own game plan for maximizing your daily function. There are skills that you'll need to develop in order to find your way through this new diagnosis-pursuing stage of your health journey. The only way I know how to build skill and ability is by remembering that it's done just *one step at a time*, while keeping your own reasons for going down this road in your full, conscious awareness. This is about changing some "default" behaviors as well as creating new habits in a sustainable way, so that you break through the stress response inherent to developing a new habit or skill.

Why evaluating and attending to daily functional ability is such a focus for me

I think about day-to-day function a lot: what it means to me and to my clients, how it changes, how it's judged, and how it's drastically affected by acute and chronic illness, disease or injury. You could say that awareness of function is ingrained in me and has been ever since I trained as an Occupational Therapist (OT) in the 1970's. Assessing the detailed impact to function or quality of life of any altered functional ability, due to mental, emotional or physical health challenges, is the mainstay of an Occupational Therapy approach.

Function is also an important part of the Traditional Chinese Medicine (TCM) view of health, which was my subsequent training and career path from my 30's to my late 50's. In TCM, as in OT, the *function* of our mind, body and spirit is intertwined and inseparable, and is affected by many influences such as weather, seasons, inherited tendencies, food, mindset, pathogens, stress, exercise, and many other factors.

My developed and trained view of how our body, mind and spirit can be affected — indeed impaired — by many divergent influences which can profoundly affect day-to-day function is a fully holistic one. Each profession I practiced had its own tools and methods, but the bottom line was always this: illness affects function. The way it affects function varies widely from one person to the next, because it will affect mind, body and spirit in ways unique to the individual. What totally devastates one person is no big deal for another.

Here's a story that comes to mind to illustrate how injury, illness or disability affects everyone differently. One of the clients I treated when I was a hand therapist taught me this lesson well. He had a severe, crushing injury to his little finger. Despite six months of rehab, he had barely regained any motion. It stuck out and got in the way and was constantly painful. He was scheduled to have the finger amputated so he could get on with work and life and have better hand function overall. It was going to make his life and his hand function much easier. Not a big choice, right? It would seem many of us would make that trade. But for him, it was a devastating choice. The surgical staff could not understand his resistance to booking the surgery that would relieve all his pain, allow him to sleep at night and to work again in his role as the family wage earner. As his therapist, I talked to him quietly in a private room to explore what was really going on. In tears, he shared with me that for the past 15 years in his marriage, he and his wife would link little fingers when they walked each evening. It was their special quiet time, their unspoken way of connecting emotionally by *that specific* form of touch as they shared their day. It was the way it had always been for them.

I realized that we health professionals err when we judge what appears to be a minor injury or procedure for another person and attempt to minimize or rationalize their reaction. He clearly needed to grieve this loss in order to choose to move forward with the surgery. Having the time and privacy to talk openly with me about the reason behind his reluctance to go ahead with the surgery helped him make the decision to proceed with the operation. His pain was then totally relieved and his hand function fully restored, minus that finger. He and his wife established a new way to connect as they walked.

In my work with clients, I have always maintained that the impact of illness or injury on all aspects of function needs to be fully acknowledged, and carefully analyzed, so that it can then be addressed in a very practical way. By increasing your understanding of how *your response to your illness*, as well as the illness itself, is affecting every aspect of your life, you have a rich bank of information available to you. By becoming aware of your conscious and subconscious attitudes and beliefs, and how they affect your behaviors and your choices of actions, you will be able to take more control over the things that may feel out of your control at this moment. You will be able to influence how you feel physically, mentally and emotionally as you navigate your way through the medical system. Identifying and shifting your unconstructive underlying beliefs and attitudes is a key process that I undertake with my clients in my life coaching practice now.

Paying attention to function was always such an automatic and seamless process for me that I confess I sometimes *forgot* that years of training were involved — that I have honed this as a learned skill. I soon realized through being ill myself that learning how to fully pay attention and to build my ability as a detached observer of *my own* symptoms, feelings, mental state and attitudes is not as easy as it appears, despite all that training! It's so much harder to see ourselves and our own beliefs objectively. It's easier to do so from the stance of an outside person. It's so automatic to get caught up in the moment, especially at times of pain and high emotion, such that your objectivity can go right out the window. That's where enlisting the help of a professional can really make a difference, and has helped me sort through my own challenges.

I'd like to share with you some important things that I've learned, that when I pay attention to them, have a critical influence on my ability to function with chronic illness. I hope my own learning will be of value to you, too.

As I've learned and thought about these skills, over many years of trial and error, I realize that they can be broken down into 3 main components. I call them the **Why, What and How of Maximizing Daily Function.**

Q #1: Why do you need to Maximize Daily Function?
A: Because you have a lot to do, and you're going to need everything you can muster up to do it.

You are faced with a big job, that of getting a difficult-to-diagnose condition properly diagnosed. So the first thing you'll need to ask yourself, and be really honest about is: *What are you doing this for, anyway?* The reason you need to be really, really clear with yourself about this is simple. The answer to this question will be your anchor in moving forward. It will be the place you will return to, again and again, when you feel like giving up. It will be your solace when life gets hard and you struggle through another dead end in your health care appointment exploration. It will be your anchor when you are too tired and worn down to do one more test, appointment or phone call, or fax one more piece of medical documentation.

What are your reasons for not just curling up in a little

ball and giving up — on your health, your life, and accepting the status quo of how your illness is now playing out day to day? *Why* do you want to look further? *Why* does it matter to you? Is this ongoing investigation being done for your own sake, or is it to appease someone else? If it's for someone else, you need to stop and take a hard look at this right now. You will ultimately need to find a reason to make it *about you*, or you may just give up when the going gets even tougher.

If it is for *you*, bravo! You have just taken the first step towards placing yourself number one on your own to-do list. You have just drawn that line in the sand and made that declaration: *"No more."* You have just found that driver inside you that you will need: the strong sense that you're doing this because you matter, because your life matters, and because you deserve more. *You* are making *your health* a top priority, because you realize that no one else can do this for you.

There may be lots of motivating factors for you that *involve* other people and relationships. You may want to vacation with your partner in a state of better health, pursue meaningful work that has been on hold, be in better shape to play with your grandchildren, or enjoy many aspects of life that have slowly slipped away in a haze of illness, pain and functional loss. But let's be clear right now: you need to be fully, unapologetically in touch with the truth that *you are doing this for yourself.*

In order to ride the wave of the health care machine, and move forward into Lyme diagnostic land, there are things you'll have to do every day to be in the best shape possible, while already ill, to take on this task. *Keep your eye on the prize:* continue to focus on why you're doing this. That's your *"why"*. Now we go to the *"what"* of maximizing daily function.

Q #2: What are the areas of daily function that you need to maximize?

A: (a) Your Habits and (b) Your Pacing.

(a) Your habits: Developing healthy habits is a cornerstone of making the most of your daily function. Why do I know this? Because I know what it's like to barely have any energy to get through all or part of a day. If I did not have a pile of well-honed daily habits, I would never have had enough brain cells left to write this book, see any clients, let alone find the energy and stamina to research my way towards finally getting a Lyme diagnosis. And I did some of each of those things at the same time, although not all of those things at once.

So what exactly is a habit? Tynan, author of *Superhuman by Habit*, says that a habit is "an action that you take on a repeated basis with little or no required effort or thought."[70] Brian Johnson, originator of Philosopher's Notes, an inspirational online personal growth and transformation platform, has summarized key learnings from numerous books related to healthy habit formation. He's really helped me shape my view of constructive habits, in terms of them being a very desirable thing to *deliberately cultivate* in order to get more of what I want out of life.

Habits are your friend. Habits make your daily activities more efficient, because they are a way of training your brain to run on autopilot through an array of routine tasks so that you can use your foggy, limited mental capacity to do the stuff that you'd really rather be doing. Once you train your brain to know "what to do when" in order to accomplish a whole bunch of day to day tasks, you will realize more time and energy for other things, and won't need to reinvent the wheel ten times a day. I have found that looking at habits from this perspective, as a favorable thing to cultivate, takes some of the sting out of the feeling that my life lacks the spontaneity that I wish was more possible because I depend on routines and habits. I have realized that it's *because* I have some good habits that there is ever anything left over — in terms of energy — to allow for *some* spontaneity of activity at this point in my early recovery process.

Here are some examples of habits that I've created in order to free up some of my time and energy:

Handling the 'body restoration basics': Maximizing nutrition, hydration, sleep and rest are crucial health cornerstones to creating the best platform possible while you are undergoing further diagnosis, as well as to have in place during your recovery. These are the fundamentals that you will always need to pay attention to, in order to build a healthier immune system so that you can deal with the pathogens and stresses from various sources that your body is attempting to process. This is one area of health care in which most camps are in agreement: these basic self-care habits are needed in order to maximize your state of health.

Exactly what a 'good' diet consists of is the subject of endless professional and popular debate. Your results are best when a highly-individualized diet, with professional guidance, is a part of your recovery plan. For the purposes of this book, I make the assumption that we all need to emphasize real foods, not processed foods, in our daily diet. You will need proper protein sources, healthy complex carbohydrates, lots of vegetables, and lots of water. You will need to minimize or avoid sugar and junk food entirely. You may need to investigate potential food sensitivities and avoid certain inflammatory offenders, such as gluten and dairy, like I do. There are lots of free and paid resources out there to help you with the many details of creating an eating plan that will optimize your well-being. I've listed some of my favorites on my webpage in Your Quick Start Guide to Unveiling Lyme Disease (your free resources are listed on the Thank You page at the back of this book).

From the standpoint of making healthy food a priority in our household, and the trial and error of preparing quality meals as quickly and easily as possible, I've adopted a few routine practices that I've found to be really helpful. They include:

- Batch cooking and freezing of meats, soups and stews in individual portions for quick meals.

- Preparing large bins for the fridge full of washed salad greens and fresh produce for several days.

- Creating meal assembly kits, made from pre-cooked quantities of healthy items like chicken, quinoa, brown rice or sweet potatoes. These are cooked in bulk and then stored in containers in the fridge, to grab easily to generate 1-bowl meals with no effort.

- Making a list of dinners for the week in advance.

- Keeping a running shopping list on the fridge.

- Getting help with the actual grocery shopping.

- Keeping a set of favorite healthy recipes in a binder, and a list of non-recipe, fast and healthy meal preps that can be done frequently, and the ingredients on hand for them.

- To keep up hydration, I keep a 16-ounce water glass on the go all the time, and automatically pack a big, refillable water bottle whenever I leave the house.

- I have a routine every night comprised of wind-down bedtime preparation, and a pre-sleep routine based on principles of good sleep hygiene.

- I have pre-set alarms on my smart phone to alert me to snack, rest, meds and nap times so that my basic daily healthcare tasks are handled and pre-dictable without using mental energy when I am not doing them.

These habits were all created for myself, but I didn't get it all right the first time. I learned what was right for me by first going through a period of trial and error. After assessing how my energy was affected by various things through the day, and noting how I responded to various changes, I'd implement a new routine and then observe the response. When a routine seemed to work, I kept doing it — until it became a habit.

What's this bringing up for you? What habits do you think that *you'd* like to cultivate to make your life easier day to day? Take a moment and jot it down!

Creating Visual cuing systems: One of the ways I've found effective to deal with brain fog and save energy is to set up some reminders visually in the house to cue me to do everyday tasks. This way my brain just sees the item and knows what to do, without my having to remember or rethink it — or spend energy thinking about it when it is not time to do that routine. For example, I have my sizable number of supplements in a bin on the kitchen counter with my master list to remind me to take them after each meal. I then pull out the ones for the next meal and line them up on the counter in front of the bin. That way, when I clear up that meal's dishes, what I need to take next is right there. I do the same on the bathroom countertop before bed, and for the next morning. Or, I will often take out all the supplements needed for the next day's meal-times dosing and place them in labeled small containers or labeled Ziploc bags, so I can easily grab them and not have to re-open several bottles each meal or pop that meal's bag in my purse if I'm going out to eat. When I take a medication as part of a long list of items or at between meal timing, I turn the bottle upside down so I remember that I took that dose and don't risk double dosing. This series of systems is fast, easy and reliable compared to having to pull out my reference sheet every time, and go into cabinets trying to remember what is needed, especially when it is a complex routine of supplements that involves products taken 5-6 times a day at specific intervals and under specific conditions (like empty stomach, or with a meal, etc.).

Priorities and list making: I've been known as the queen of sticky notes. I must admit that the copious use of sticky notes and list-making has allowed me to live a busy and productive life at home and when working during many years of chronic illness and variable levels of function. On days when my brain has been mostly mush and my emotions are on overwhelm, the use of lists and sticky notes for dealing with every facet of my day has kept me focused and served to calm me down. I combine list-making methods, meaning I use both paper and electronic versions of reminders, depending on the task. There are so many time management systems available that can be learned and used. The important thing is to develop some kind of basic organizational strategy — and use it all the time. The more you can get things out of your head and onto paper or electronic screen, the more energy it frees up for your brain to use on thinking about other things.

Setting and frequently re-adjusting priorities is key to managing limited energy and the variability that can occur with Lyme symptoms or other chronic illnesses. What is most important to you in the grand scheme of things? What is less important, or can be delayed until you feel a bit better on another day? Remember how important it is to keep your eye on the prize: is this set of activities you're doing today bringing you closer to finally getting a diagnosis and solving your health care issues? In his book, *Only 10's*, Mark J. Silverman describes how focusing daily on what really matters to you, the day's '10' — then trusting your inner knowing to guide that process — is really the best answer to greater results and productivity in creating what you want out of your life.

Managing supplement regimens: One of the things

you'll likely encounter in a holistic recovery program from chronic illness, including Lyme disease and its related co-infections, is the need to take a number of supplements to augment your health. This may already be a part of your daily life now. The use of natural products for health enhancement and symptom relief has been one of my primary methods of treatment for several decades. I had to find a way to streamline my system of tracking, ordering, assembling and taking supplements (and for a time, prescription Lyme medications), such that it was not a constant strain, mix-up or taking excessive time. The system that I've adopted has consisted of making a versioned Word document with my name and lists of supplements, and it is organized by time of day taken, name of supplier, name of product, potency (e.g. 250 mg) and dosage. I now order everything from three main online suppliers monthly and have them delivered. I adjust the list with any new practitioner recommendations, and I can readily print a copy to take to any medical consultations. I use very tiny Ziploc bags that we buy from a local industrial supplier for single mealtime, bedtime etc., doses for travel.

(b) Your Pacing: the other key component of the 'what' for maximizing your daily function.

I've found a surprising amount of 'sneaky stress' that happens — in my own experience and that of clients — when dealing with medical appointments, evaluations, and health care decisions. Trying to incorporate a significant amount of health care activity, such as that involved in researching and pursuing diagnostic help, can be truly exhausting. It can trigger a roller coaster of fear, excitement, hope, disappointment, and frustration. Sometimes even the simplest of tasks can turn into hours of red tape, waiting, being on hold, endless phone calls and bureaucracy. Sometimes what appears to be a great option–and finally the answer you've been seeking — doesn't work out for some reason.

The path to diagnosis will take you a lot of places — physically, mentally and emotionally — that are uncomfortable for you. Expecting yourself, and your family if you have one, to just incorporate all of this extra time, stress and activity into a 'normal' daily life in any kind of seamless fashion can be unreasonable and unfair. Already, your life has likely been severely disrupted by illness, or you wouldn't be reading this book. To expect to add a few more notches of activity and intensity without some kind of daily adaptation is unrealistic.

Energy conservation as a practice is your cornerstone of self-care. When your energy gas tank is only half full or less to start with, you need to avoid the emptying of that tank in order to protect your precious physical, mental and emotional energy. You can think of this as your energy bank account, and it is important to realize it has no overdraft protection.

Becoming energy-aware is a skill that takes some practice and constant self-awareness. What are the circumstances, people and activities that give you energy, and what are the ones that take it away? Remember, what stresses you may not stress someone else to the same degree, or vice versa. You need to see what that is for you, and adjust your daily and weekly timetable accordingly. On a week that you have more medical appointments or health care preparation activities, you may need to schedule more quiet time alone for self-care, or more emotional support with a friend, coach or counselor. Keeping a few written, dated notes in a blank journal is a simple way to start noticing trends about how your energy level and key symptoms respond to different stressors and stimuli.

Watch for medical system overload challenges. Scheduling and spreading out the tasks involved in appointment preparation, such as your long medical history or supplement list update, can help you better cope with those tasks. As you undertake each of the steps towards getting a diagnosis, the reality of your health situation will strike you in various ways at various times. This can be emotionally exhausting to process — being faced with truths that you may have thought you knew, yet had not experienced them in such a stark way as when confronted in a medical setting, for example, can be a surprise if it is not expected. You need to allow time and space and self-kindness for all of this to unfold, as it needs to. Remember it is part of your emotional healing to lean into this discomfort as you learn to deal with it. This is one way to reframe having a hard time — remembering that everything that happens is somehow in support of your ultimate goal. Again, recalling your why is also crucial to staying centered at times like these.

You can pay attention to your own body's cues to help you decide when you can 'afford' to push through to complete a task, vs. when you may be better off taking a break from appointments, testing, research and decisions for a few days — or even weeks. If in doubt, take a break, give yourself the opportunity for some laughter or a good book or movie, get a night's sleep and come back to your task the next day. Your body's stress regulation systems will be glad that you took a breather.

Q #3: How do you Maximize Daily Function? By Cultivating Self-Awareness and Nervous System Resilience

The intricate interconnections between your mind, body, emotions and nervous system are vitally important to work with on your path to improved health. Your mind and emotions will often seem to present you with difficulties, stubborn resistance, painful realizations and amazing "Aha" moments. These complex aspects of yourself contain the potential for more untold power and infinite possibilities than you may ever have imagined. *That's why these interconnections present both opportunity and challenge.*

Those with chronic illness know that navigating your way through your health journey can mess with your mind and emotions in ways that those without chronic illness cannot even begin to appreciate. This topic of mental and emotional health is so vast and so dear to my deepest curiosity and passion, that I feel like I could write many books on this topic alone with what I've learned so far. And that would be just barely cracking the surface! There is more on the importance of attending to mind/body/emotional connections and approaches as part of your healing journey in Chapter Five.

I'm going to attempt to narrow down some of my key learning so far into some basic, practical tips that relate your mental, emotional and nervous system awareness to *maximizing your daily function*. What are some of the key skills that you can develop in order to cope with the demands of daily life in a more productive, authentic and self-aware way while moving along your diagnostic path and into recovery?

Cultivating your Observer Self is a key step in being able to stay relatively objective in the face of emotional turmoil during your health care journey. It means learning how to keep a part of your mind able to notice, in a neutral way, what you are feeling, thinking and doing. It means being aware of your body and attuning to its many varied sensations and feelings, without being so overwhelmed by them that you find you just cut yourself off from noticing anything beyond your busy mind and its endless, often worried thoughts.

Compassionately and neutrally observing yourself means you can avoid "just running on autopilot" or — at the other end of the spectrum — being overpowered by intense emotion. When your observer self is 'on', there will always be a part of you that can sense what is truly happening in any given scenario. This observer part can hold a place of steadiness, authenticity and self-acceptance that simply is not present when you are mindlessly engaged in the routine activities of life and automatically going through the motions, or simply reacting to the stimuli of your day.

The reason it is so important to learn how to strengthen this observer part of yourself is that it can be your friend, monitor your feeling state, and notice what is going on, so that you always have a pulse on what is *really* happening within you. It is a place of non-judgment and of full presence and being, not of *doing*. It is a place from which you can build your self-awareness so you can then take specific actions that allow you to enhance your own body's innate healing.

So how do you cultivate this 'observer self' further? If this is a brand-new concept for you, you may also wonder what the heck I'm talking about. How can you be feeling or doing something, and watching yourself do it, at the same time? This is something that has to be experienced to be understood.

On a very basic and important level, being more aware of the state you are in and how you are feeling physically and emotionally (rather than being so caught up in your present experience that you are not able to really 'observe' your state) involves having a healthy and resilient nervous system. This takes specific learning and practice.

Your autonomic (automatic) nervous system is responsible for the fight, flight and freeze response, as well as diverse physiological body processes (e.g. digestion, heartrate, breathing) and your capacity for joy and human social connection and engagement. It is highly affected by your family history, your upbringing, and your life-long experiences of physical, mental or emotional trauma. This trauma may originate from many different sources and be judged as being of varying degrees of intensity — but all degrees of trauma can be significant.

There are many ways that your nervous system can be thrown into fight/flight states of uncomfortably high or prolonged stress chemistry, and into a freeze/shutdown state that renders you exhausted and mentally/emotionally numb, among other adverse symptoms. Lack of regulation of the nervous system — for example, by staying in a state of physiological stress for extended periods, or in a state of prolonged shutdown — directly affects your immune function, among other significant body processes. This has a direct bearing on the development of illness, as well as affecting your recovery from chronic illness.[71]

The inter-relationship between the state of the human nervous system and emotional, physical and mental health is well-recognized by many who work in the field of trauma therapy — for example by highly regarded trauma therapist and author Peter Levine, founder of Somatic Experiencing.[72] Unfortunately, despite its critical importance, the effect of trauma on the nervous system and on your overall health is not yet well acknowledged or treated in mainstream health care, let alone in our own day to day living.

The well-quoted 1998 article on ACE (Adverse Childhood Experiences),[73] a study done on almost 14,000 subjects, showed a direct correlation between early childhood trauma and the development of significant illness as an adult. Trauma has dramatic, lasting effects on the human nervous system and directly influences our reaction to and recovery from stressors throughout our life.

What can you do to ensure that you are building up your 'observer self', so that your overall health can benefit from this heightened state of self-awareness? A common method that has been used for millennia to strengthen the observer self is through various forms of meditation. There are countless meditation resources available now in-person and online, easily accessible by a quick online search.

The only caveat I would mention here regarding meditation, is that if you have had early life trauma or even trauma as an adult, I would recommend that you first begin with a good nervous system education and regulation program. This will help you to improve your self-awareness about the varying states of your nervous system and to learn specific tools to strengthen your nervous system resilience. Diving directly into a meditation program when you have a history of unresolved trauma may be problematic — or at least less than helpful.

Why do appropriate nervous system education or trauma therapy approaches provide important groundwork to make your meditation practice more enjoyable and successful? The typical aspects involved in meditation of being able to be aware of and more comfortable with sitting quietly and reflecting inward, and noticing your body's sensations, are not necessarily comfortable if you've had trauma and are used to living only in your head. For example, you can find yourself more anxious and agitated (even lasting beyond the meditation session) instead of the anticipated state of calm. You may even start to blame yourself for a reaction that is not your fault (i.e. because your reaction is due to your trauma history's influence). Then you may come to the false and frustrating conclusion that you are a failure at meditation — or even worse, mistakenly believe that you may never be able to learn how to relax. It may just be that you are using the wrong tools in the wrong order.

You need to first be able to tune into yourself in small,

comfortable increments, and develop a deeper, body-felt understanding of how you can positively influence the health of your nervous system. It takes specific, slow, repetitive and guided practices to build greater stress capacity and nervous system resilience over time, with specific body-awareness tools used as important groundwork. A great place to start is with the unique online materials and programs from Irene Lyon: www.irenelyon.com. I have found her material to be of huge benefit to me. She has written about how trauma adversely affects your ability to successfully participate in mindfulness meditation and other similar practices, in her blog post, *Why Mindfulness Practices Don't Work — Learning the Groundwork to Meditation*.[74]

Learning more about your own background, what trauma really means for you, and how its effects have shown up in your nervous system to influence your way of being in your life, is a key starting place for recovery. This will help you cope better with your many chronic illness stresses — as well as hasten your path to overall physiological healing.

You may be surprised to learn how much of your day is spent in fight or flight mode, taxing your adrenals and affecting your immune system due to prolonged, elevated levels of stress hormones. Also, it can be a shock to learn how often your body goes into a self-protective shutdown mode, which may appear calm on the outside, but is not a true state of healing and can interfere with your immune system function, gut healing and many other important functions. I've included some extra reading on this subject in the resource page at the back of this book.

Meditation comes in so many forms and methods. In its simplest form, for example, one way of meditating is to simply stop, close your eyes (if that is comfortable for you), and take a one-minute pause, just focusing on and noticing your breathing. Feel it, be aware of it. That's it. That's a good start. You could do this many times a day. When stressed, upset, foggy or overwhelmed, pause and notice your breathing. Notice your feet on the floor and your seat in the chair. Just start with whatever simple practice feels most comfortable to you.

When you learn how to live more of your life with your observer self 'on', by learning about your nervous system, working with it in gentle, targeted ways and being able to build better stress resilience through body/mind/emotion awareness, it will change your life — and your health.

Self-care and self-acknowledgement is your antidote to the martyr or victim trap. Let's face it, we've all been there: those times when living with illness sucks so much that you can't stand another moment of it. You want to escape, but there's nowhere to run, because your mind and body keep following you *wherever you go*. You feel hard done by, alone, miserable and may decide that no one understands how difficult it is to go through it all. You see others out there enjoying their lives and the freedom they seem to have without dealing with major health challenges, and you can't even stand to talk to anyone. When it feels like life is closing in on you, that is a prime indicator that your energy tank has gone close to or below empty, and you need to fill it up…now! You'll need to determine what activities and situations are restorative to your mind, body and spirit. It might be a shower, a rest with a soft blanket, a warm cup of tea, or a good movie. Put it into action ASAP…that means now!

Deliberate positive input is a key way to soften and quiet down your brain's innate survival response. Our brains are actually wired to look for danger and to perceive threats. So, left unattended and to its own devices, when threatened by illness the brain will continue to look for all kinds of danger and alert you to be on guard. This includes anything new, different, or uncomfortable — like, say, pursuing a Lyme diagnosis! Knowing that this is how your brain works, that it's normal, and *is going to happen* can be a distinct strategic advantage. It means that you know you'll need to find ways to calm it down and replace the stimuli that it perceives as dangerous with at least some other things that will be perceived as 'safe.'

As mentioned previously, working with the nervous system in strategic ways to help modulate a survival response that is too easily triggered is essential. Ways of bringing a sense of safety to your physiology is especially important if you have a history of trauma.

Positive input can often be perceived as 'safe', because it can be temporarily distracting, engaging and can divert your attention away from thoughts that ramp you up. Instead, your attention is placed onto something that feels more nurturing, interesting or helpful. This can be a useful resource to support your physiology, helping to reduce adverse or prolonged manifestations of the fight, flight or freeze aspects of your survival response.

You can deliberately use positive input to rewire new areas of your brain to produce feel-good chemistry. Examples of this may be favorite music, or downloadable audios and videos that are uplifting, funny or empowering. When I made the conscious decision to start my day with a short, positive personal growth video on my tablet at breakfast, I began my days with a whole new state of mind that carried me through many a harrowing health care predicament. (Thank you, Brian Johnson, for your inspiring *Philosopher's Notes TV!*)

Gaining control and knowing how to surrender: It may seem strange to talk about both control and surrender in the same sentence. They seem to be opposite concepts, but yet they can coexist. There is a certain duality of attitude that I've found helpful to adopt here. That attitude has taken me a long time to develop (and is still a work in progress). It is one that encompasses both surrender and non-resistance to the way things are (i.e. you are sick and have some significant symptoms) as well as an attitude of taking action or control over the things that you really *can* influence to help you feel better as you're going through all of this. Both surrender and action are important elements to your journey — and each is a choice that you can actively make on your own behalf.

Playing with this concept of surrender and control can help you create a feeling of greater self-acceptance while still moving yourself forward to get the help you need by taking strong action. By assessing how various external stimuli and activities affect you, you can learn how to better recognize what you do and don't have control over. This then allows you to make the most of your fluctuating energy levels, especially knowing you will need to adjust by manipulating or compensating for outside variables. For example, if the activity you had planned for a certain day feels like too much, you may need to limit its length or learn how to set only tentative plans that may have to be postponed at the last minute if your energy level or symptom set does not support doing them after all. *Flexibility without guilt* can be a valuable attitude to cultivate.

The dark days: Handling the days when life just sucks can be a big challenge. There are times when you just feel like giving up and succumbing to staying sick forever, because the effort of getting help just doesn't feel like it's worth it. These are the days that really require you to practice intensive self-care. These are signals that you have tapped that finite energy bank way too much and must make some specific efforts to refill it. Learn how to recognize your own signs of overwhelm before they get too severe, so that you can alert yourself to the need for extra self-nurturing. Pushing harder through these tough times just doesn't work.

What are the signs that show up for YOU that indicate you're going down this slippery slope towards darkness and meltdown? Is it irritability, worsening insomnia, wanting to chew out anyone who looks at you sideways? Does it feel like everyone in the world is suddenly an idiot, personally bent on making your life miserable? Does it seem like you are suddenly very alone, that living in the world is impossible, and you need to run away because no one can possibly understand you? Does your appetite go way up or down, or your digestive system go wonky? Do you feel more brain fog, dizziness, or lightheaded? Does your pain level go up? Do you feel like you have PMS on steroids? (That's my all-time favorite indicator that I need to practice self-care first aid). Learn to recognize your own set of warning symptoms that you've gone past your internal threshold of tolerance, so that you can take action to remedy this imbalance before it escalates further into full meltdown.

One of my favorite resources for learning more about practicing self-care is Cheryl Richardson's book, *The Art of Extreme Self-Care.* She describes the necessity of implementing radical self-care to prevent illness (let alone how important it is when you already *have* illness). Her ideas about developing a self-care 'first aid kit' prepared as a checklist for yourself to use in times of crisis are really helpful. You will then be able to turn to it at any time, especially when your energy has really tanked, so you don't have to re-think who to call and what to do in order to calm yourself down and take a restorative physical and mental rest.

Sharpen your communication clarity: Being honest with yourself is one of the skills that you may think just goes with the territory of being human. We're all honest with ourselves, right? After all, what's the point in lying to yourself, when it's "only" your own mind that will know the difference?

Well, there are all kinds of reasons that you may have trouble feeling what you really feel and acknowledging what is really going on inside your own mind. And that is akin to lying. Not deliberate lying, more like lying by omission. This is due to all kinds of internal censoring that you may be really good at doing at this point, because you have been conditioned to find what you're feeling or thinking "unacceptable." And if you can't be fully honest with yourself and own up to what's really going on, then any embarrassment or shame that accompanies your own thoughts will also get in the way of communicating your needs to others.

So why does this matter? It can get in the way of communicating important information with your health care providers, because you're too embarrassed and self-blaming to say how you feel, and you may therefore under-report symptoms, or distort your picture of functioning, when in a discussion that could make a difference in their recommendations. It can get in the way of communicating with your spouse, family, or friends, and contribute to a downward spiral of loneliness, disconnection and misunderstandings in the context of your relationships. It can get in the way of others offering you much-needed support, because they don't understand the full picture of what you're really going through.

Remember my stories in Chapter Two, along the theme of how I soldiered on for so many years, pretending I was OK in order to just keep going in my various careers? That behavior cost me a lot of potential support from extended family and friends, because they didn't have a clue what was really going on. Looking back, I know that I could have had more caring and tangible support shown to me, but I was not able to let it be known how I was really feeling. In fact, I couldn't even let it be known to myself.

Learning how to be fully aware and honest with

yourself is a skill. It doesn't just happen by itself. It takes courage, persistence, practice, and often the help of a coach or trauma therapist to see what obstacles are in the way, so you can eliminate them, or at least be aware of the impact of them. This is one of the key areas we focus toward in my in-depth work with my one-on-one and group coaching clients. Self-integrity can free up and enhance your relationship with yourself and others in amazing ways that you may not be able to imagine, if you have yet to experience it.

Honing your core values: Another piece related to shoring up your mindset and emotional state relates to getting clear on what your values are. If someone asked you right now, "What really matters to you, and why?" What would you tell them? Would you be able to snap off a few values that you live by, that you refuse to compromise as you deal with various health professionals and medical scenarios? Would you have to think about it? Or would you struggle to articulate them?

What values are you expecting to be shown by others in the way that they treat you, yet you don't show to yourself? If you want to be treated with honesty, fairness, kindness and respect by your health professionals, how are you showing these values to yourself first? Becoming more consciously aware of what you hold most dear to you, and how this influences your behavior towards yourself and others, can be an important realization. We can't expect others to treat us in ways that we don't yet know to treat ourselves, or practice treating ourselves. If you treat yourself with respect and kindness, the energy that carries forward from this will also affect how others treat you.

Understanding how your increased personal value awareness influences your decisions can be used to your advantage. It informs what you will and won't tolerate. This can help your decision-making, such as the hiring and firing of certain health team members. Certain decisions could then be more confident no-brainers for you when they are clearly aligned with your values, rather than based upon vague impressions or just an uneasy sense that you aren't getting what you need. When your strong personal values are violated, the ensuing stress will let you know very clearly who you want to have in your life and who you don't. This applies to everyone from the health professionals to whom you entrust your care, to the people in your circle who you want to be a bigger or smaller part of your new life as you recover.

No matter what, you're still you: The experience of being ill for so long, and having to find your way in the medical system, offers so many opportunities to get very clear on the inner workings of your own mind. But awareness of these opportunities is often lost because you can readily become mired in a sea of miserable physical symptoms and emotional feelings. It's so common to experience helplessness, fear and powerlessness in the face of so many medical investigations, endless appointments, and at times having to deal with insensitive or unhelpful attitudes from others. There is a lot to react to, if you are in a reactive state.

At times when I could finally step back in that self-observer role and breathe a little, I discovered some ways to help myself with these all too common feelings that I, too, experienced. I became well aware of what constant exhaustion and other multiple symptoms of chronic illness would, and did, take away from me: my careers and business successes; my finances; my social life and some of my family and friend relationships; some of my pleasures, hobbies and interests; a lot of my independence; my faith and hope at times; and my trust in my own body's capacity to heal and to be able to be relied on to function every day. The grief of these losses for all of us with significant health challenges is very real.

But then I began to look at the things that chronic illness *can't* take away from anyone and *hasn't* taken away from me. Chronic illness could not take away my values. *What really matters to me and why it matters will always be a part of who I am.* My anger, righteousness and indignation, sparked over the many years of medical system navigating and significant health challenges, served to fuel my positive values of justice, fairness, honesty and kindness. These positive values have now been honed to a razor-sharp edge. The strengthening of these kinds of values, that you may be noticing in yourself also, are potent fuel for advancing your skills of self-advocacy in navigating the medical system.

Another choice that can't be taken away from you is *where you decide to place your thoughts and attention.* I realized over time that where I focused my attention indeed remained my own choice, and this was always true, at any given time. I learned different ways that I could capitalize on this ability of focused attention and set clear intention to positively influence the outcome of many situations. This focused attention skill training will serve you well in all areas of life… for the rest of your life.

The other remaining thing that could not be taken away by illness was my innate survival instinct. That remained fully intact, and it did its very best to serve me well and protect me. The stimulation of your basic survival instinct has so many implications in your ability to function. Although its very important job is to keep you alive, I learned that the survival brain's hyper-responsiveness to stimuli can also be at the root of many of the symptoms encountered in any chronic illness. Although you very much need your innate instinct to survive, you also have to learn how to keep it from getting over-aroused to the point that you are locked into fight/flight/freeze response too much of the time, at the expense of turning on your body's tremendous self-healing energy. I'll be addressing more about this important topic in Chapter Five.

The navigating of life with chronic illness on any given day, while simply trying to function in the world, is a feat in itself. You are braver than you may realize. Remember that at any given time you are doing the best you can. That's all we can ask of ourselves. Showing yourself that extra kindness and compassion as you continue to find your way through further self-growth will go a long way. It will help the overall recovery of your sense of personal pride and will fuel your gradual reentry into the world of better health and higher activity level in a very powerful way.

Chapter 5: Acknowledging Mind, Body and Spirit Connections
Skill # 3: Build Greater Self-Awareness to Facilitate Your Recovery

"…everything can be taken from a man but one thing: the last of the human freedoms — to choose one's attitude in any given set of circumstances, to choose one's own way."
— *Viktor Frankl, Man's Search for Meaning*

You may have reached a point, this far in your health journey, where you feel broken. You are likely worn out by it all. The thought of having to find a place within yourself to dig deeper for more answers, let alone embark on a new, potentially prolonged treatment course, if you do have chronic Lyme disease, is intimidating. If you have read this far in this book, you have reason to believe Lyme could be the mystery you have been looking to solve. However, that doesn't mean that you're comfortable with the idea of facing the many internal layers of self that pursuing a new diagnosis will unveil.

Some thoughts to consider

There are two things that I feel are critical points for you to consider as you move forward from this exact place.

First, I want to let you know that no matter how down-trodden you may feel, you are not broken. Your spirit is alive and well, however it may seem to retreat somewhere deep inside you. Your immune system innately knows what to do to help you get well. This reality will seem clearer when you give it the support it needs to do so. This support can come in multiple forms, from traditional medicine to alternative and complementary therapies, even mind-body-spirit modalities. Everything that supports well-being can support your immune strength.

Second, you can't splinter off any part of yourself and deal with it in isolation, whether it be a body part or a body system, or your mind. I believe that we are all divine beings and are all part of a greater whole. Just as we are interconnected with each other and the whole Universe, your mind, body and spirit are inextricably linked within your living human reality. They were not separate when you got sick, they are not separate now, as you work on getting a definitive diagnosis, and they won't be separable when you embark on whatever treatment you choose.

Whatever your choices for your ongoing health care management, in order to fully navigate and recover from any health challenge, I believe that you need to fully embrace a holistic view of health and function. My experience, both professionally and personally, has led me to this belief system. Without these experiences, I would not have developed the clarity and skills that I've been describing and sharing with you in this book. Alongside my own health struggles for many years, whether because or in spite of them, my passion for my continual learning about well-being, through a variety of lenses, has never stopped.

From orthodox medical science to the fascination of the intuitive and energy world, to say I've experienced a lot is an understatement…and it all has shaped who I am today. A self-professed skeptic, it's taken a lot of first-hand experience for me to fully embrace the world of energy and intuition. Indeed, I have only done so by concurrently maintaining a consistent grounding in science.

I used to think I had to make a choice between one and the other. Then, to my relief, I gradually realized that left-brain analysis and right-brain perception are not really separate ways of knowing anyway. They are not mutually exclusive. They are part of a continuum. Another continuum is the form by which the body, the mind, the spirit and the realities of Universal energy and matter interconnect, some of which our senses do not seem to readily understand. The tools and methods for discernment on the surface appear to be separate. Each has its specific strengths and applications.

A medical doctor, trained in allopathic medicine, uses drugs. A holistic practitioner may use herbs. A massage therapist uses touch. A life coach uses words. Whether consciously aware of it or not, they all use intention, energy and spirit alongside trained knowledge and tools, and they all bring exactly who they are to the healing process when they interact with you. And all of it affects you in turn, whether you fully realize it or not. Call it science or call it woo-woo…. or acknowledge both. It's just how energy works.

The influence of energy on healing reminds me of an interview I saw from Oprah Winfrey on her *Super Soul Sunday* TV program with Dr. Jill Bolte Taylor, which aired July 26, 2015. Dr. Taylor is the author of *My Stroke of Insight*, and a neuroscientist who suffered a massive stroke at age 37, resulting in her entire conscious function being reduced to a right-brained, intuitive awareness. The left hemisphere of her brain, with its reasoning, logical function was completely offline. She described being acutely aware of the energy of each person that came into her hospital room, whether they were a staff member or someone with whom she had a personal relationship. The presence of someone's energy was all she could understand, because the usual way of relating and understanding, with words and concepts, was totally lost to her during that time. She recounted the compassion of one physician who, instead of condescendingly talking over her or about her as if she wasn't there, spoke kindly, clearly and directly to Jill. But the message was in the energy, not in the words, which were unintelligible to Jill at the time. She later said of the physician, *"She recognized that I was wounded, not stupid."*[75] This intention made a tremendous difference in enhancing Jill's ability to heal, as it created within the challenging hospital environment an atmosphere of kindness, caring and trust. The energy we allow into our world when dealing with our health issues really matters.

Harnessing the Power of your Immune System to help you

When you have a chronic illness such as Lyme, something has gone wrong in your immune system in the first place–that allowed this to happen at all. As mentioned in Chapter One, so many things can stress the human organism, and finally there comes a tipping point when the immune system becomes overwhelmed.

Our mind and body are connected in countless ways. There is a direct association between stress and immune system function. The long-term release of excess stress hormones such as cortisol can contribute to inflammatory conditions and then suppress the healthy immune response that is needed to fight pathogens.[76]

Adrenal fatigue is a common issue with chronic illnesses. Responding to various types of chronic stressors, prolonged cortisol release as in the case of recurrent fight or flight response will eventually create adrenal dysfunction, with its own set of troubling symptoms — such as fatigue, anxiety, depression, insomnia and digestive disturbances.[77]

Combinations of factors such as pathogens like Lyme and its common co-infections, past and current (often cumulative) physical and emotional life stressors including trauma, environmental pollution, nutritional issues and the like can strain your immune system to a point where it is no longer effective. Even the emotional stressors of living with chronic health issues themselves can further compromise one's immune system function, creating a negative spiral. Autoimmune diseases, such as rheumatoid arthritis and lupus–conditions that have been seen in the past as random occurrences by orthodox medicine — are now recognized within the functional medicine model as manifestations of inflammatory processes from various causes. These diseases occur when the immune system goes haywire, resulting in the body attacking its own tissues.[78]

The immune system is a complex, wondrous, functional marvel. More is discovered every day about its inner workings, and how it interconnects with every other system of the body. How the brain works, to oversee and referee the trillions of processes that occur every second in our bodies, is nothing short of miraculous.

So much is happening within us that is presently under the radar of our conscious awareness. We have just begun to learn to tap the incredible potential of what our brains, with the proper kind of training, can do to influence all of our body systems and functions. The profound changes that can occur in a state of health and well-being, with focused mind intention and specifically chosen techniques, have moved from the fantasy of science fiction to today's quantum physics reality.

In Chapter Four I introduced the notion to embrace both surrender and control as you navigate your health path. While surrendering to the reality that you have work to do in order to pin down your diagnosis and enter into new treatments, I want to give you a sneak preview of some of the ways in which you can influence your state of health and well-being, even without having that specific new diagnosis yet in hand. This applies to you now, as you are involved in focused diagnostic work, and literally for the rest of your life.

Why a Lyme Diagnosis matters

I believe that getting a diagnosis of Lyme disease and any related co-infections will change your life. Knowing what you're dealing with brings tremendous mental and emotional relief. There is finally a *reason* for so many symptoms you have suffered for so long, which to date have not made sense. It can also feel like a relief because it seems that you now finally have a specific target for medical intervention. Here is a known pathogen that responds to various pathogen-killing measures. This creates an initial sense of satisfaction in the human psyche: *I know what the enemy is, and now I'm going to get my weapons and kill it.*

The way you live your life finally has a change in focus: from struggling or managing to eke out a meager survival and adaptation of your life through adverse, puzzling, and often misunderstood symptoms — to clear attention towards a goal. That can feel really good for you and for your loved ones.

It's Complicated

But there is also a conundrum. The simple approach is limited. *Let's target this pathogen and kill it and everything will be fine* just won't cut it with chronic Lyme. There is too much, systemically, already going on. First, the ways in which this pathogen is medically treated are not simple, black and white approaches. There is also a lot of discrepancy of professional opinion on the most appropriate medical treatment.

And the reason why you are sick with Lyme in the first place is a multifaceted picture. That reality of immune system complexity, with all of its inherent mind-body-spirit connections, applies to Lyme with full force. In order to recover, I am convinced that you will need to adopt a holistic approach.

I struggled with writing this chapter, because this is a book about finding your way through the complexities of getting a Lyme diagnosis. So why am I now talking about treatment and recovery issues? Because the reason you want a diagnosis in the first place doesn't just stop at getting a diagnosis. You're doing it because you want to get well. I get that. I also didn't want to mislead you into thinking that as long as you get a diagnosis, then you're home free. Then the hard work would be all done. That narrow attitude, *"Just identify and kill the bugs,"* goes fully against all of my 40 years in health care, both as a professional practitioner and as a patient.

During my initial training and professional experience as an occupational therapist in the 1970's and early 1980's, the lens through which I viewed health and illness was limited to the allopathic medical model. I simply didn't realize what else was available, and there was much less readily accessible at that time, compared to the present day of exploding growth in holistic health care. The presence of the internet has also profoundly changed the face of health care options and access. As a therapist, I began to notice the wide discrepancies in patient recovery, despite standard treatments being applied to similar conditions. Some deep and troubling questions emerged for me: given the same disease or condition, what were the factors that made one person recover well, yet another still remained sick or disabled? Why did some treatments 'fail' while others 'succeed', for what appeared to be the same condition? What made one person have such a positive attitude throughout their rehab process, while another failed to respond and stayed in a state of victimized misery? What was the secret to motivating someone to do what it took to follow therapy instructions, exercises, and recommendations to get well?

I began to search further for answers through my own personal growth path, as well as through embracing long term studying and practice in various holistic healing paradigms and modalities. This included everything from reiki and therapeutic touch to Traditional Chinese Medicine and acupuncture, to other forms of intuitive and energy medicine-based healing. As my information base grew, I witnessed my patients and myself getting better results using a holistic model. My attitude continued to broaden. After a time, there was no looking back. I simply could never again embrace the Western medical model as an *exclusive* path to health recovery.

Your Recovery can start while pursuing your Diagnosis

I knew I had to address *what's next* here, because holding a vision of where you're ultimately going — and what you'll need to know and do to be successful — is important. Remember how I talked about keeping your eye on the prize of getting a diagnosis, so you can wade through all those steps? Well, it's also important to keep your eye on the ultimate goal: *your wellness*. And to get there, you're going to need to look beyond the pathogens. So why not start now? Knowing some of the options that are available to you can catapult you into recovery, as well as make your health issues during your diagnostic slogging somewhat easier to cope with.

There are other things that I think really matter toward your overall wellness, that go far beyond pathogen killing. These are things that no matter what your final diagnosis, Lyme or not, and how much time passes in the meantime during your focused diagnostic journey, you're going to need to address at some point in order to fully get well. These include some (possibly surprising) factors that may have affected your tendency to get sick in the first place. When addressed, making changes in these areas will help you no matter what.

These changes have to do with your brain, your nervous system, your energy, your state of mind, and your spirit. They are wellness elements that go far beyond bug killing but are not separate from bugs or their destruction. It's all connected because *you* are all connected.

Let's look briefly at some of the considerable knowledge and techniques available in mind-body medicine these days. These are topics that you can choose to study further as a way to strongly influence your state of health no matter what your diagnostic outcome, whether Lyme and co-infections or not.

Beyond Bug Killing: Holistic models in Health care

Earlier in Chapter One, we looked at the some of the strengths and limitations of the Western medical model. Having experienced both western and eastern models of medicine and practice, from both a professional practitioner standpoint as well as a consumer/patient standpoint, you can imagine that I have developed some strong opinions. And my current view is this: each system has something to offer. And no system is complete or perfect. This reality that there is no one-size-fits-all solution to health care issues has spurred the emergence of relatively newer models within modern medicine, such as Integrated Medicine and Functional Medicine. But the concept of holistic care is not new. It is the backbone of some the oldest health care systems: Indigenous Medicine, Chinese Medicine and Ayurvedic Medicine.

In my own health care journey, I have assembled and reassembled various health care teams for diagnostic and treatment purposes, based on my variables that ranged from practical issues such as geographical access and financial realities, to the matching of philosophical approaches. We all have to find our own way with these complexities, myself included.

There are Lyme treatment specialists, and extensive online and written resources that I have found in my search so far, in every discipline from Chinese medicine and acupuncture to Homeopathy, Naturopathy, Integrative medicine, Bio-individualized medicine and Epigenetics, Nutrition, energy and spiritual healing approaches and more. Each of these models has merit, differs in how the client is assessed, and varies in the tools and methods employed for treatment. Description of these vast resources is beyond the scope of this book.

The main point of discernment about these approaches, relative to the strict Western medical model, is that inherent in the approach is taking a holistic view of the client. All of these fully integrated health care systems look at the contribution and interconnection of mind, body, and spirit to the state of wellness or dis-ease in the individual. As well, there is account for the role of environmental factors, pathogens and similar external influences, viewed in the context of all these interrelationships.

All of the holistic models that I have checked out also use a medical Lyme and co-infection diagnosis as valuable information. Despite some of these models using their own unique diagnostic methods, language and labeling techniques, a Western medicine-based Lyme diagnosis is considered to be an integral part of the holistic picture and a relevant insight. That leads me to the belief that having a Western medical diagnosis of Lyme and co-infections is still an important advantage, even when pursuing healing through other, non-Western approaches, models and systems.

How over-activation of the survival response can affect your entire state of health

Our brain is wired first and foremost for survival. What survival truly means is effectively responding to life and death situations in an adaptive manner. We can and do automatically protect ourselves by fighting, fleeing, or freezing/shutting down in the face of threats or extreme stressors. The physiological and anatomical parts of the brain and nervous system that are key to this important mechanism include the brain stem, the limbic system, (which consists of a set of structures such as the amygdala, located deep within the center of the brain),[79] and the vagus nerve (one of the 12 cranial nerves emerging from the brainstem). The vagus nerve is an important structure that connects with various internal organs and tissues in the neck, chest and abdomen. It affects many autonomic nervous system (automatic) functions in the body such as breathing, heart rate and digestion. It also influences our ability to socially connect with others, perform some sophisticated brain functions and engage our innate, regenerative healing systems.[80]

In the case of chronic illness, the brain's survival responses tend to be over-reactive. There are many different reasons for this, but all paths have led to one core problem: dysregulation of the nervous system.[81]

The reasons for this dysregulation are physiologically-based, comprised of one or several of the following factors: environmental assaults that stress the body, such as toxic chemicals or heavy metal exposure; pathogens such as Lyme and co-infections, that cause inflammation and raise cortisol levels; various physical, mental and emotional stresses (including early trauma); and the expression of genetic predispositions that have been triggered by physical and emotional stressors. Even significant biochemical influences, stemming from trauma suffered by your family's previous generations, can be a factor affecting your health and influencing illness.[82]

The marvelous, life-saving automatic survival response runs awry in your physiology when the brain interprets acute or cumulative non-threatening stimuli as life-threatening. This easily reactive, inappropriate, misfiring over-responsiveness is beyond our conscious control, *but it can be retrained*, due to a phenomenon known as neuroplasticity. This well-studied observation is that the brain has an essential and innate ability to rewire itself in response to new, consciously-placed input, in order to behave in new ways.[83, 84]

What are the signs that you may have nervous system dysregulation? This is where it can get both complicated and amazing. Many of the signs of nervous system dysregulation are *the same set of systemic signs and symptoms that occur with common chronic illnesses*. These illnesses include Lyme disease and co-infections, chronic fatigue syndrome, fibromyalgia, MS, POTS, multiple chemical sensitivities and various autoimmune diseases. Some of these symptoms include fatigue, brain fog, pain, depression, irritability, oversensitivity to sights, sounds, smells, or electromagnetic stimulation, anxiety, blood pressure fluctuations, headaches, heart palpitations, gastrointestinal issues, sleep disturbances, and many more. As you can see, it can become difficult to determine which symptoms are pathogen-related and which ones are nervous system dysregulation-related.

Neuroplasticity: the brain can recover and can influence the body's healing

Although the model of neuroplasticity is very well-researched, well-documented and active in clinical practice, its application to the treatment of chronic illness such as Lyme disease is still not well recognized by the mainstream medical community. This is another example where exciting, and very effective, non-medical programs exist to help people who have chronic illness such as Lyme, but it's very unlikely you'll hear about them from your MD. Chances are, you will be the one informing your MD about how well you're doing based on the programs that you have chosen! Remember, your MD is focused on application of the tools that their education promotes and trains them to use, that are sanctioned by their professional guidelines for practice. This means their insight comes from laboratory testing, trials of drugs, and surgical intervention. This mind-body work is beyond the scope of most conventional medical practices at this time.

If you're interested in studying this further, there are many fascinating books that discuss basic concepts and practical application of the principles of neuroplasticity. I have compiled some of these in a resource guide on my webpage.

Some specific approaches to brain/nervous system and body healing: Nervous System Regulation, Advanced Cell Training (ACT), Dynamic Neural Retraining System (DNRS), The Gupta Program (amygdala retraining), EMDR, Heart Math, EFT (Tapping)

Our brains and bodies are complex and require a multi-faceted, integrated approach to heal. Pathogen-killing is not adequate to sustaining well-being when you have a history of complex, chronic health challenges.

Here are a few examples of what is currently available and easily accessible online. I encourage you to learn more on these topics, so you can find a program and/or practitioner that may be a good fit for you.

Irene Lyon (www.irenelyon.com) has combined key knowledge and tools from the fields of body-awareness-based practices of Somatic Experiencing (founded by Peter Levine, https://traumahealing.org/about-us/), the Feldenkrais Method (founded by Moshe Feldenkrais, http://www.feldenkrais.com/moshe-feldenkrais), Somatic Practice (developed by Kathy Kain, http://www.somaticpractice.net/trainings/), and Polyvagal Theory (developed by Stephen Porges (http://www.stephenporges.com/). Applying her own science-based education and extensive client experience (both from her previous research and ongoing private practice), Irene has developed extensive online educational programs for promoting nervous system awareness and self-healing. Her broad knowledge and deep passion about nervous system physiology and the effects of trauma as it affects health and illness is outstanding. By understanding and rewiring your nervous system with methods you can use in your day to day life, you can learn how to directly modulate your body's stress responses. You can learn how to better comprehend and communicate with your own body's signals and needs, and how to release stored stresses and trauma. This can vastly improve your immune system's ability to fight pathogens, promote healing of adrenal and digestive issues, and reduce the negative physiological and emotional effects of past trauma, to name just a few of the extensive benefits available to you. This kind of neuroplastic healing takes time and patience, as you are rewiring potentially a lifetime of adverse physiological stress responses that have contributed to your illness — often in ways that you may not have been aware of. It is well worth every step. Irene's nervous system regulation programs have become an integral part of my own healing and daily practice. I highly recommend including this as a key aspect of your healing journey.

Yet another holistic approach to healing on a profoundly deep level is *Advanced Cell Training*, ACT (www.advancedcelltraining.com/ACT). This brilliant, proven approach was developed by founder Gary Blier for healing chronic Lyme disease and other chronic illnesses. This innovative approach uses a unique system of specific energetic principles, working at the cellular level to retrain the body to restore physical and emotional health. Gary developed this program after healing his own severe chronic health issues, using creative and solid applications of his extensive knowledge of holistic healing modalities. ACT's clinical success specific to chronic Lyme disease is well-documented by its enthusiastic participants https://www.facebook.com/pg/AdvancedCellTraining/ reviews/?ref=page_internal). This program has been one of my key choices in my own path towards healing from chronic illness and I highly recommend it.

There are also some limbic system-based neuroplasticity programs that you may wish to explore. These are based on the premise that since so many symptoms in chronic illnesses are associated with heightened activation of the body's innate survival response (i.e. fight/flight/freeze), you need to approach healing from the perspective of calming down the brain's inappropriate and overactive response to stimuli and retrain a new response These well-organized and results-oriented international programs offer at-home participation via online access as well as instruction through in-person training. These include *The Dynamic Neural Retraining System* (www.dnrsystem.com), developed by Annie Hopper, and the *Gupta Program*, an amygdala retraining program developed by Ashok Gupta. (www.guptaprogramme.com). There are many testimonials online attributing excellent recovery to these programs. Each program's founder recovered their health from serious chronic illness using the program they developed.

One caveat I would like to offer is that if you have had a history of any trauma, a nervous system regulation-based program and/or 1 on 1 trauma therapy with an experienced therapist is highly recommended as a critical starting point for deep, effective healing in order to deal with the many complexities that come up with this type of personal background. And remember, as I mentioned regarding the ACE study on Chapter Four, a trauma history is very common in people with chronic illnesses of various kinds.

You may think that what you have experienced is not 'trauma' if you weren't overtly physically or sexually abused as a child, for example. But trauma can be understood as anything that overwhelms the nervous system or is beyond its capacity to physiologically handle, and can include a wide range of life events.[85, 86] This broad definition can explain to so many people why they are not getting the results they think should be happening with countless medical and therapeutic interventions. Even the brain rewiring/limbic system-based programs like those mentioned above may require some trauma healing work as an important base. Dealing with your early trauma by accessing skilled support is a must for overall healing. Time is not enough in itself to heal from past trauma that is held in the cells of the body.[87] If your body has been living a lifetime being on 'high alert' within your nervous system, true healing needs to include strategically tuning into the body and helping the nervous system to build renewed capacity for handling stress. Your physiology needs to learn how to feel a new level of safety.

Eye Movement Desensitization and Reprocessing (EMDR) (www.emdria.org) is another approach that is very effective at rewiring brain function and addressing stored stress and trauma in order to promote effective overall healing. This well-researched and very effective treatment uses protocols that have been developed from a range of original treatment approaches. It can be found as one of the specific methods used by certain licensed therapists. It has been another one of the key tools I have used on my own recovery path.

Another physiological healing approach is *Heart Math* (www.heartmath.org), which helps re-train the heart-mind connection for calming purposes and relief of stress-related symptoms such as insomnia, anxiety, and fatigue, which are also often seen in chronic illness.

EFT (Emotional Freedom Technique) http://www. emofree.com/eft-tutorial/tapping-basics/what-is-eft.html or 'tapping' is another simple yet effective method used successfully by many people to help resolve mind-body concerns. Many articles cite the reduction of diverse symptoms of chronic illness using this method.[88] Information is widely accessible online and guidance is readily available through many holistic healing practitioners.

Fight, Flight, Freeze/Shutdown: How your survival brain protects you from perceived danger

The specific response of the survival-oriented brain to a perceived danger can present in a variety of ways from stressor to stressor, and person to person. The powerful responses of fight, flight, and freeze or shutdown can be very obvious and overt, or they may show up much more subtly in various behaviors and symptoms. The perceived stressor may induce anything from severe anxiety to total life-threatening collapse due to blood pressure and breathing issues, to an uncomfortable sense of irritability, a spacey feeling, inability to think clearly, and even avoidance of eye contact in a personal situation that feels confrontational.

Something as general as chronic fatigue can therefore actually be caused by a complex interplay between a response to childhood trauma, a nervous system over-re-action due to adverse biochemical influence from pathogens, an immune response to the pathogens themselves, and an ensuing freeze/shutdown response. So, the recognized, 'physical' cause of the fatigue may be only one of the key players, along with the very real and often dramatic automatic responses to various subconscious and physiological triggers.

Here's a personal example related to my own relentless chronic fatigue. As I worked through some of my own aspects of nervous system triggering, and what was labelled as PTSD based on childhood issues, I began to notice that a portion of the severe fatigue I had experienced for so many years was actually the result of cumulative and early stresses, leading to a repetitive shutdown response. The response would hit me suddenly and without my conscious awareness as to why. At times, I could barely hold myself up in a chair, as it took all I could do to stay upright and functional. This had happened to me for many years, while I tried to track and figure out all kinds of reasons for it, focusing on physical ones such as food sensitivity reactions or over-doing it, activity-wise. As I worked through many aspects of my symptoms using EMDR and other techniques with a therapist who excels in treating trauma response, I began to realize that many of my Lyme symptoms — including severe fatigue, and neurologically-oriented symptoms like dizziness and vertigo — were further complicated by my trauma history. I was experiencing a strong shut-down reaction, not 'just' fatigue related to an inflammatory response to pathogens. Even though the physical aspects of

Lyme and other co-infection bacteria and viruses remained real contributors to my fatigue, I began to understand that some of the triggers for my feelings of shutdown in day-to-day life had to do with trauma. I have continued to work on ways to resolve these patterns using various nervous system regulation and energy healing techniques.

It can take a talented health professional, body worker or therapist, who is well trained in trauma healing methods, to help you discern and treat any significant early trauma aspects influencing your health. Complications from trauma occurring later in life, such as medical trauma from dealing with many difficult facets of chronic illness, will also greatly benefit from professional support. Nervous system education and self-regulation, such as the material offered in programs provided by Irene Lyon (www.irenelyon.com), as previously mentioned, can be a very valuable starting point, if you believe this is a part of your personal profile.

The frustrating thing with complex chronic illnesses such as chronic Lyme disease—for you, as a patient, and for your doctor as well — is that despite using long-term medical treatments of various kinds, some symptoms may persist. If you don't know where to look for more answers, that can be a significant stumbling block. Again...*bug-killing may not be enough.*

It is important to note here that *this discussion does not mean that any particular symptom or response that you have is 'all in your head' or that you have or should have conscious* control over what is happening within your body. *The problem is in your physiology.* It is the underlying fact that some of your symptoms can also be related to excessive activation of *an innate survival response* that is relevant. Only methods that can access both your subconscious mind and your body — and retrain your brain and nervous system's internal wiring — will be effective to change this. You just can't over-ride this with your rational mind and use your frustration-fueled willpower to make it stop. The brain's strong survival response will always try to trump your conscious thoughts, so you have to learn to work supportively and awarely with your body's physiology rather than trying to just overpower it with your mind.

Working in *specifically structured and very gentle ways — with repetition* — to gradually shift your triggered reactions and responses will empower a new way of being. This is the basis for the various nervous system regulation, energetically-based treatments and brain rewiring programs that I have mentioned. Neuroplasticity means change is possible. It does not mean that this strong survival patterning is something you can randomly shift on your own without some kind of professional guidance and a consistent, structured program.

The lack of medical, allied health professional, and human service professional training around assessment and treatment of early trauma and your hyperactive survival responses can create a complex and puzzling situation — both for them as well as for you as a client. This makes it difficult for all concerned to detect what is actually going on, and that lack of awareness complicates your ability to find more comprehensive and effective assessment and treatment for all aspects of your chronic illness.

The field of trauma research and clinical practice is rapidly growing, but as in other areas of health care, it's challenging for professional training, especially continuing education for practitioners already in the field, to keep up with this significant growth in cutting-edge information. The professionals who are leading the way in these areas often come from fields of social work or counseling, body work, psychology and psychiatry. If you are fortunate enough to find a healing professional who is well-versed in current trauma research and practice, this can be a huge piece of solving the puzzle of your multi-symptom chronic illness.

Do you have a history of physical or emotional abuse or early trauma? Sensitive exploration, with the help of a well-trained trauma specialist, can be a huge and invaluable support to your healing. Adding energetically-based mind-body treatment processes to help you deal with the way this may be affecting your brain, nervous system and immune system now may make all the difference in your recovery. Reach out and get the help you need. You're worth it.

How chronic illness and lack of a firm diagnosis can create or aggravate a vicious cycle of nervous system dysregulation

Many far-reaching challenges inherent in living with chronic illness commonly plague those who are pursuing a possible Lyme diagnosis. This may be the case for you, too. The social and emotional traumas of an undiagnosed or mislabeled condition alone may include dealing with countless medical tests, navigating a health care system that may not be at all sympathetic, and pursuing medical interventions that turn out to be either ineffective or the cause of various uncomfortable or even serious side effects. Grief associated with the substantial losses of life roles, finances and health also presents a significant ongoing challenge.

Many people who don't yet know they have chronic Lyme disease are ridiculed or dismissed by health care personnel when they do not fit a clear diagnostic category. Rather than continuing to investigate, these professionals may pronounce that they can't find anything wrong, implying that nothing is actually wrong. All of this can wreak havoc, emotionally and mentally, on even the strongest of individuals. There is also fear that we won't recover; fear that we must be just imagining a condition because it is so elusive to name and comprehend; fear that the latest new treatment approach (for whatever the new hypothesis may be) won't work, *again*. We rapidly lose faith in our bodies' ability to function and lose hope in having the capacity to heal. We can feel helpless and powerless, despite many attempts to understand what is wrong and despite having already taken countless steps to improve our health.

Cumulative trauma, or even PTSD with its associated adverse effects on the brain and nervous system, can result from repeated losses and chronic illness stresses such as those just mentioned. It does not have to be a single huge, life-threatening event that triggers nervous system dysregulation. Intense fear and helplessness can be felt repeatedly when dealing with many 'ordinary' aspects of the medical system and various chronic health challenges.

Peter Levine, PhD, an eminent researcher, clinician and

author in the area of trauma and Body-Psychotherapy, says, *"Trauma occurs when we are intensely frightened and are either physically restrained or perceive that we are trapped. We freeze in paralysis and/or collapse in overwhelming helplessness."*[89]

One of the functions of the innate immobility — or freeze response — in mammals is to numb the terror and pain of a physical attack (e.g. as when attacked by a predator). The freeze mechanism may cause one to feel as if outside of your body, or as if what is happening is actually occurring to someone else. This subconscious distancing or dissociation function is a protective one. It helps the fear or pain to become more tolerable to you. Past trauma can create a feeling of not being safe to feel sensations and emotions in your own body. However, when dissociation becomes a frequent, patterned response in the brain and nervous system, it can have a negative effect on your day to day life. You can feel isolated from others and be unable to feel some of the normal pleasures of living life. The automatic freeze/dissociation response can even trigger various symptoms that mimic the condition you are trying to treat, such as fatigue.

This is just one example of how your intricately wired, survival-oriented brain has far-reaching implications in how you and your body will respond to the various stresses of chronic illness. Unconstructive, yet automatic feedback loops in the brain and body can complicate your recovery process, and these can add more cumulative stress to you during your medical procedures and appointments. When you feel a disproportionate amount of fear, or experience a spacey or disconnected feeling during medical interventions, the stimulation of this kind of innate survival response may be a contributing factor.

This automatic, protective dissociation response can create that sense of spacey disconnection even when you are actively trying to concentrate at a medical appointment. This can make your appointments more difficult in a very practical way. The stress of *yet another* appointment, and your desperate but as yet unmet expectations for help, can become another trauma trigger. Operating automatically from the primitive level of the survival brain can make it harder to think straight in your health care appointments, causing you to make mistakes when talking about your history or symptom reporting, to feel confused or to not retain the information provided to you.

This further complicates the very real cognitive challenges associated with the neurological complications of Lyme and co-infections. That's another reason why in Chapter Four I talked about some practical suggestions such as having organized, written systems in place to handle all of your information and your appointment questions and reports. It's not your fault. It's just another indicator of the complexity of your brain's function, the results of brain inflammation, and the far-reaching but unconscious effects of the triggered survival response. But it's important to remember that you have more control than you may think over your daily state of being. You can have a strong positive influence upon your cognitive and emotional challenges by learning more about how your nervous system works, strategically building nervous system resilience and adapting how you prioritize and manage your daily tasks.

This is another example of building up your level of self-empowerment by taking charge. You can access key resources, in order to learn and apply new information and strategies to influence your level of day to day function.

The field of early trauma and PTSD research and treatment — including medical trauma — is an extremely complex one, with important findings being newly discovered and documented. I've listed some resources for you on my webpage if you're interested in doing further reading.

Experiencing Yourself Well: Recovering lost hope through specific visualization processes

The use of creative, positive visualization as a tool for powerful personal transformation is well-documented. There are countless resources available on this subject. Some of the common features of effective approaches include deliberately creating heightened positive emotion while in a relaxed brain wave state. You need to create an experience in your mind that feels so real that your brain experiences it as if it's happening in present time. A regular positive visualization practice even initiates the wiring of new pathways in the brain. There are many amazing published accounts of people who have completely changed their state of health and totally changed their life through intensive and repetitive daily visualization methods. They have learned how to consciously affect their subconscious mind, creating a new way of being in the world.[90]

Sounds like a great idea to do this, right? But when you have an exhausting chronic illness, the thought of adding *one more thing* to your daily regimen, even something positive like a targeted visualization program, can be enough to make you want to hurl something at whomever suggested it. I've been there. And your perceived ability to visualize a new positive reality for your life may have gone completely down the drain, along with your dashed hopes for answers and recovery after yet another dead-end medical consultation appointment. You may be struggling just to get through another day. I've been there, too.

When your physiology is in a survival state of flight/ flight or freeze, the function of the parts of the brain responsible for higher cognition such as positive visualization is not 'online' to be readily available to you. I've observed and experienced that this can be a common occurrence in times of distressing relapse of your illness, or when you're under an extra load of emotional or physical stress. The necessity to be able to deliberately tune into heightened positive feeling states can be very difficult during these times. So, don't beat yourself up for not being able to 'do it right'. Particularly if you have a history of trauma, as mentioned in Chapter Four, understand that you may need to start in a much gentler place of establishing basic nervous system safety first and gradually build comfort and skill in tuning into your body and your feelings.

In the many attempts I've made over the years to pick myself up again and try yet another new thing to get well, I've immersed myself in a number of different methods and programs involving guided meditation, visualization and positive outcome creation. I've experienced varying degrees of success, but despite many months at a time of dedicated daily practice, the improved health outcomes I was hoping for did not seem to last. In retrospect, based on the number of approaches I've tried, I realize that I needed to do further groundwork on supporting my nervous system first, due to the early trauma and adult medical trauma I've experienced. This may be the case for you, too. Don't underestimate the power that an early trauma history has on your life as an adult and its role in chronic illness. It doesn't just resolve itself with time. It needs to be addressed with specific methods.

My positive personal experience with Irene Lyon's materials and her unique 12-week group program (www.irene-lyon.com), as well as what I've witnessed in my classmates' progress, has led me to believe that this is the best place to start if you've had a history of any early trauma, medical trauma or are dealing with the common fight/flight/ freeze responses of chronic illness. I believe this gentle, foundational work on understanding and improving nervous system health is the cornerstone to better health. It is an effective, gradual route to brain rewiring. It can help you achieve a better state of mind, a heightened and more comfortable connection with your body, enhanced acceptance and expression of emotions and improved physical health. It's the non-medical program that has helped me the most so far to reduce my stress and anxiety, cope better with difficult medical issues or procedures, and intensify my self-compassion. It has given me a range of effective, simple tools for daily practice that I truly appreciate.

I'd like to recommend one thing to you: *keep trying to address your brain and nervous system issues, and don't give up!* If you don't resonate with one particular program or mentor, then try another one until you find a good fit. Attending to our mental/emotional/energetic state is critical to managing the stresses of chronic illness and to building a solid health recovery plan.

Deep acknowledgement of your humanity: vibrational transformation, breathing, presence

In my quest for larger meaning in my life, and seeking recovery of the parts of myself that I felt had been so lost in the sea of chronic illness, I've come across a few important resources, available both in-person and in written or experiential program form.

One of my dearest, most influential mentors in recent years is Panache Desai, who describes himself as a spiritual thought leader and a catalyst for vibrational transformation. The energetic presence that comes through in his interactions is unique and profound. One way that he helps people who are engaging in deep personal change and transformation is by eliciting an increasing conscious awareness of some very basic, yet profound realities. The key ways I have *understood and experienced* some of these realities is as follows. Please note that this is my own interpretation based upon my experience in my work with Panache:

- We are all spiritual, infinite, Divine beings here on earth having a human experience.

- Our ultimate purpose here is to love and be loved.

- The world needs each one of us: our uniqueness, our contribution.

- Nothing about our experience here or about us is bad, wrong or a mistake. We can't screw up. It is all just learning and experiencing.

- Our life experiences are driven by our soul's mission and our Divine connection; we can make plans, have goals, but ultimately our soul will play out its path that we came here to do. We can either resist that or we can learn how to receive and embrace it.

- All pain comes from resisting what is.

- As any strong emotion arises, breathe and let it wash through you. It is our willingness to feel and to be who we are that will transform us.

- We might as well enjoy the adventure of being human.

- It's all, ultimately as well as right now, OK.

I have presented this information as food for thought here, because I believe that having a mentor or a set of guiding spiritual beliefs can help us recapture our authenticity. Whatever our starting place, a deeper connection with our own authenticity frees us to live in a way that reduces stress and allows us to reach our potential by re-igniting our purpose and passion. The need for finding deeper purpose, based on who we truly are, is aligned to my own professional roots in Occupational Therapy, where it is understood that engaging in purposeful activity and paying attention to mind, body and spirit is critical to human wellness and recovery.

It's not your old life you're getting back. It's a new one.

"But in those moments when disappointment is washing over us and we're desperately trying to get our heads and hearts around what is or is not going to be, the death of our expectations can be painful beyond measure."

— *Brené Brown, Rising Strong*

Even in recent years, I used to think that promising my clients something like how to "Get Your Life Back" would be what people wanted and some version of that would be what I should aspire to as a good coach. That's what everyone wants, right? To go back to your pre-sick days, to full recovery, to the things you used to do and the way you used to live. The pre-sick days can become kind of glorified as the mental, emotional and physical 'crap' that you have carried around, often unawarely, can get lost in the wistfulness of reminiscing.

I am going to deliberately burst your bubble, and ask you to reconsider the notion that returning to the life you used to have is *really* what you want. I'll explain. That "wanting my old life back" bubble spontaneously burst for me, yet the process was so gradual that I didn't realize until much later that it had even happened.

What I learned is this: the way I was, my usual way of being and doing, was *what led me to getting sick in the first place.* The energy implicit in the ways I thought, felt, lived my days, and the conversion of that energy into the physical matter of my body and my immune system (combined with a crapload of early life trauma, stresses and external 'bugs'), is what created the perfect storm that overwhelmed my system. I got sicker and sicker. It turned out to be Lyme and its co-infections that comprised my most recent and specific target for medical intervention. But maybe if not for those pathogens, my story could have been cancer, or MS, or something else. Was it just my unique combination of factors that led to this particular illness cocktail? Likely we will never know. It dawned on me that *going back to who I was no longer remained a viable option...* not if I wanted to create a new, healthy body and a renewed, vibrant life.

Inadvertently, the things I have explored and the changes I've made in my conscious and subconscious mind and nervous system have gradually created a new me — that's a good thing. To the outside world, I may look the same, except for some weight gain thanks to my illness and some more grey hair. I may even be seen as more ambitious, and less patient, in some ways, while more patient or accepting in others. I may be not so accommodating. I may be just a tad more outspoken. Well, *maybe a lot more.*

But inside, I can feel the changes and they are profound. My 'bullshit tolerance' is just about nil. That means I am far less capable of tolerating any crap — from myself or from others. My urgency to *stop* making myself small, and instead to step up, get out in the world and make a difference with what I've learned and what I know, has burned a hole through my soul! And I may be *even more* bursting with love and more desiring to show it to others. That is because I am finally full of more love and respect — for myself.

This whole process has changed me, too. Getting a

medical diagnosis that explained so much of what I had gone through health-wise, gave me a deep acknowledgement that I had been craving for several decades. In spite of my initial reluctance, I believe that using several different antibiotics to kill the Lyme and co-infection pathogens was an important contribution to my ongoing recovery. It was through finally getting the Lyme disease and co-infections diagnosis and applying a targeted treatment that all of the self-help, supplements, diet, energy work, lifestyle modification, holistic healing and exploration that I'd been doing for a lot of my life — and continue to do now — have had a chance to really take hold. I know that I'm on my way into bigger recovery now.

This has been a slow process and an ever-evolving one. I believe I will always be a 'work in progress', and some days, it's still not pretty — physically or emotionally. When it comes to the evolving of my own awareness and consciousness, the working through of my 'stuff', I'll never be 'there'; I'll never be 'done'. *I don't think any of us ever are.*

As you continue on your health journey, parts of the old you will remain true to who you will always be: your spirit, your values, the essence of what you love, what drives you forward, and what makes you tick. At the same time, a part of you will necessarily die. You can't go through a major health crisis, or any crisis, and emerge as the same person who entered that crisis. Crisis changes people. Whether you acknowledge it or not, it has already changed you. *How this change manifests in your day to day life and how your level of consciousness evolves as a result is something that you can influence in profound ways.*

What kind of a new life do you want to create? How do you want to live? How do you want to feel? It's up to you. So much is possible.

> *"Patients cannot believe that their chronic illness will*
> *continue and embrace change simultaneously."*
> — *Annie Hopper, Wired for Healing*

> *"Action is the antidote to despair."*
> — *Joan Baez*

Conclusion: Lost No More

Lost

I am lost.

I don't know who I am.
I don't know what I am doing.
I don't know where I am going.

Somewhere in the darkness I see
the flickering flame
of a tiny candle.
But it is so far away.

There is a hand
reaching, reaching,
reaching out to me.
But I cannot quite grasp it.

I feel a soft, warm breath on my shoulder
but when I turn around,
no one is there.

I know what I must do.

I must run faster and faster after that dim light
until its brightness dazzles my eyes.

I must stretch to meet that hand
until it is firmly clasped in mine.

I must whirl around to face
that Being, close behind me.

But all this takes courage,
time,
patience,
and perseverance.

It is much easier to simply sit down and say:

I am lost.

Lisa Dennys, 1967

* * *

I wrote this poem when I was 12 years old. It came to me as a kind of divine vision; like a download, experienced before home computers were a part of life and that term was ever invented, whether applied to information obtained from a network of machines or a spiritual realm.

I remember it clearly. I just walked over to my desk in my bedroom, and I wrote it down all at once, not really thinking about it, just delivering the message onto a piece of paper. When I was finished, I read it and I tried to figure out what it meant. It felt really important. I kept it, although my twelve-year-old self didn't fully understand. This poem has guided me through my whole life to this day. I have come back to it again and again. At many significant times in my life I've re-interpreted what it really means to me, and what it is here to teach me about.

Now I realize this poem is about really seeing the guidance and help from both human and divine sources that have always been there for me. That help was there for me, even when I could hardly see it, or when it seemed impossibly far out of my reach or especially challenging, given my circumstances.

It's also about my shadow side, my darkness, my fear and my feeling-not-good-enough self, the self that I have always sensed was breathing down my neck and taunting me, that I was too afraid to turn and face. Now that I have faced her, she is really not so scary after all. It's about grit and about stepping into personal power and what it takes to do that. It's about how easy it is to just say it's all just too hard, to simply give up.

* * *

However far you've come in your journey back to health, I applaud you. You are here reading this book because you are still looking for answers. You have not given up.

You can choose to view your experience this far in many different ways. It has been hard. It's still hard. And you will continue to have some challenges. That's how *life* is.

Writer and filmmaker Jonas Elrod, in his personal growth program on Oprah's OWN TV network, called *In Deep Shift*,[91] chronicles the moving and diverse stories of people who've gone through very significant life events. Through the lens of these individuals' journeys, he talks about three discrete self-transformation stages on our spiritual path, each of which we may go through when encountering any deep life crisis. These stages are *Breakdown*, *Breakthrough*, and *Integration*.

The *Breakdown* stage is summed up as: "...when the floor drops from underneath your feet."[92] This is when we encounter and are knocked down by huge obstacles in life including personal crises and significant losses, accidents, injuries or serious illnesses. Life as you knew it has ceased.

Breakthrough is characterized as your defining moment, the one when you realize that you actually have a choice about how you are going to proceed in your life. It can be a do-or-die kind of dramatic decision, or a slower-moving, yet significant kind of epiphany. It is the time when a deep shift in your awareness has occurred: we sometimes call this your "Aha" moment. You realize that your life has been forever altered and that you need to reach deep inside of yourself to create something brand new out of your personal tragedy.

The stage of *Integration* is the one in which all the magic of spiritual and personal transformation fully manifests. Now that your life has been forever changed by what you have gone through, and you realize that you need to live in a different way, it's time to create that new reality. This is when you make sense of what has happened, and you choose to look at it from the perspective of who you are now, and how this experience has changed you. You embrace the deeper learning that has occurred. It's when you realize you will never be the same, and at some level you're OK with that. Possibly more than OK with that, maybe the experience has yielded some really positive changes, to be celebrated regardless of how difficult their entry into your life may have been.

It's this *Integration* stage that really interests me, because I have seen so many people who don't quite make it this far. This stage requires a *decision* to spend effort in conscious processing of what's happened to you. I've worked with many patients and clients, in my own professional journeys, who have chosen to embrace their health crisis head-on and do the considerable self-exploration work required to emerge personally transformed. Their bodies may or may not be healed to varying degrees, but their minds and spirits have come to a place of ever-evolving deeper peace and self-acceptance. In fact, I believe that *not* integrating what has happened to you so far, and staying within only the first two stages, is kind of a cruel joke against your own humanity. You're missing out on the richness and deep sense of peace that your life's path can offer you.

In my own journey, I can say that I am still in the process of Integration, and maybe that will go on forever. I don't know. I do know that the many years of illness, the losses, the getting up and starting over again (and again) have deeply affected who I am, and how I view everything. I know that I have had to make several key decisions that reflected my desire to truly live, instead of settling or giving up.

I want you to know that your life is worth living, even on the days that it may feel too bleak and too tiring to bother anymore. I want you to know that you can find more answers, and that help is always available to you. And above all, that you don't have to do all of this alone.

Ruling Lyme disease in or out, once and for all, is a very worthwhile endeavor, so that you can get on with the process of getting better and living fully. I have the confidence in you that you will find the resources that you need — both inside and outside of yourself — to make this happen. I know that your diagnostic task ahead is daunting, and can feel overwhelming.

Here's my summary of the factors that I believe will influence your success in making your way through your medical and personal journey towards getting a diagnosis. Remember these short statements as your mantras through each stage of the road ahead and know I am traveling it with you, however short distance ahead I may have gone.

- Make your health and getting a clear diagnosis to solve your health puzzle a top priority: *You are Number 1*!

- Use the guidelines in this book to research online

and choose key health care practitioners with the *wonder quotient*.

- Continue to build and refine your health care team, during the phases of diagnosis and treatment, as you sharpen your medical system navigation skills.

- Pay attention to your daily energy level, and rhythms of day-to-day life, and adjust what you need to in order to maximize your energy. This alone will help make some of your symptoms more tolerable.

- Learn what both surrender and control mean to you, and how tension and the dynamic between the two plays out in your life, in your health and otherwise.

- Identify and strengthen key internal and external resources; ask for help with whatever is realistic to allow you to focus on your wellness for now.

- Cultivate an attitude of self-acknowledgement and self-acceptance as you build a new life that reflects who you really are and what matters most to you.

- Pay attention to your spiritual self and find ways to nurture it.

- Learn how to trust your own decisions about what is right for you at every step as you navigate your unique health journey. Your own inner knowing, intuition, and experience are all valid tools to use in negotiating your own path.

I hope that the information and encouragement that

I set out to provide for you in this book have given you a helpful place to start.

Do You Want Some Further Help?

I want to give you a couple of ways to move forward from the material presented in this book.

Here are two options for you:

- **You can choose to work with me personally to guide you through this process.** It's a tough road to navigate out there! If you're new to online investigating of the most appropriate health care resources for your own unique needs, it can be a challenging, lonely and overwhelming task. Hiring the best, key health care professionals, and navigating your way through the learning, skill development and inner adjustment processes of your journey back to health takes a lot of effort and know-how. I get it. I've been there, and had to learn how to find my way through this difficult process when I didn't even know where to start. If you'd like some expertise and guidance on your determined path to better health, and you want to get there as quickly and efficiently as possible, I can help. This link will take you directly to detailed information about how you can get support from me as your coach: www.unveilinglyme.com/workwithlisa.

  You can also email me at: info@unveilinglyme.com.

- **You can access some further complimentary resources here:**

  Please go to: www.unveilinglyme.com/thankyou to download my free resource package for readers, *Your Quick Start Guide to Unveiling Lyme Disease.*

Endnotes

Introduction

1 http://www.aapsonline.org/liegner/IOM-Letter.pdf

2 Katina I. Makris, *Out of the Woods: Healing from Lyme Disease for Body, Mind and Spirit* (New York: Helios Press, 2015), 253.

3 http://www.cdc.gov/lyme/stats/humancases.html

4 http://www.cdc.gov/hiv/statistics/basics/ataglance.html

5 http://www.cdc.gov/cancer/breast/statistics/

6 http://www.cdc.gov/cancer/colorectal/statistics/index.htm

7 http://www.healthline.com/health/multiple-sclerosis/facts-statistics-infographic

8 http://www.ilads.org/lyme/lyme-tips.php

9 http://articles.mercola.com/sites/articles/archive/2012/02/05/dr-dietrich-klinghardt-on-lyme-disease.aspx

10 http://articles.mercola.com/sites/articles/archive/2012/10/13/under-our-skin-documentary.aspx

11 https://en.wikipedia.org/wiki/Chronic_fatigue_syn-

drome#cite_note-CDCBasic-12

12 http://www.myfibro.com/fibromyalgia-statistics

13 http://articles.mercola.com/sites/articles/
archive/2012/10/13/under-our-skin-documentary.aspx

14 Richard I. Horowitz, *Why Can't I Get Better? Solving the Mystery of Lyme & Chronic Disease* (New York: St. Martin's Press, 2013), 28, 155

15 Ibid., 163.

16 http://www.ilads.org/lyme/about-lyme.php

17 http://emedicine.medscape.com/article/330178-clinical

18 Richard I. Horowitz, *Why Can't I Get Better? Solving the Mystery of Lyme & Chronic Disease* (New York: St. Martin's Press, 2013), 23

19 http://med.brown.edu/neurology/articles/sr21608.pdf

20 http://www.cdc.gov/lyme/signs_symptoms/lymecarditis.html

21 http://www.idsociety.org/uploadedFiles/IDSA/
Topics_of_Interest/Lyme_Disease/Policy_Documents/Lyme%20Disease%20Testimony-Global%20Health%20Subcommittee.pdf

22 http://www.cdc.gov/chronicdisease/

23 http://www.ccgh-csih.ca/assets/Elmslie.pdf

24 Ibid.

25 http://www.idsociety.org/uploadedFiles/IDSA/
Topics_of_Interest/Lyme_Disease/Policy_Docu-

ments/Lyme%20Disease%20Testimony-Global%20
Health%20Subcommittee.pdf

26 http://www.ilads.org/lyme/about-lyme.php

27 http://www.cdc.gov/lyme/diagnosistesting/

28 http://cid.oxfordjournals.org/content/43/9/1089.full

29 http://www.lyme-disease-research-database.com/chron-
ic-lyme-disease.html

30 http://www.casewatch.org/board/med/burrascano/
order.shtml

31 Jess Armine, Blog Talk Radio Show, *POTS...the 411!*
February 2, 2015 http://methylationsupport.com/dev/
podcasts/

32 http://www.ilads.org/lyme/about-lyme.php

33 http://criticalhealthfacts.com/dying-of-lyme-disease-
case-fatality-rate-nearly-100/

Chapter 1

34 http://www.epatientdave.com/2013/03/10/source-
for-17-years-for-new-medical-practices-to-be-adopt-
ed/#comment-224210

35 http://www.ct.gov/dph/cwp/view.asp?
a=3136&q=388506 A Brief History of Lyme Disease in
Connecticut

36 http://www.lymeneteurope.org/info/the-difficul-
ty-of-culturing-spirochetes

37 http://www.ilads.org/lyme/about-lyme.php

38 http://articles.mercola.com/sites/articles/
    archive/2012/02/05/dr-dietrich-klinghardt-on-lyme-
    disease.aspx February 05, 2012.Why is Lyme Disease
    Not JUST a Tick-Borne Disease Any More

39 http://lymeontario.com/about/about-lyme-disease-2/

40 Middelveen MJ, Bandoski C, Burke J, Sapi E, Mayne
    PJ, Stricker RB *Isolation and detection of Borrelia Burg-
    dorferi from human vaginal and seminal secretions.*

41 https://www.health.ny.gov/diseases/communicable/
    lyme/fact_sheet.htm

42 Alison W. Rebman , Lauren A. Crowder, Allison Kirk-
    patrick, John N. Aucott *Characteristics of seroconversion
    and implications for diagnosis of post-treatment Lyme
    disease syndrome: acute and convalescent serology among a
    prospective cohort of early Lyme disease patients.* Clinical
    Rheumatology March 2015, Volume 34, Issue 3, pp
    585-589   http://link.springer.com/article/10.1007/
    s10067-014-2706-z

43 Shawn Bean, Blog Talk Radio Show, *MTHFR & Meth-
    ylation Awareness,* Oct. 17, 2013. http://methylation-
    support.com/dev/podcasts/

44 http://canlyme.com/just-diagnosed/testing

45 http://www.health.gov.on.ca/en/ms/lyme/pro/

46 http://www.health.gov.on.ca/en/public/publications/
    disease/lyme.aspx

47 Jess Armine, Blog Talk Radio Show, *Lyme Disease: the
    411!* June 23, 2014.

48 Lesley Fein, Shawn Bean, Jess Armine Blog Talk Radio

Show, *Lyme Disease: Open Mic Night: Time to ask the Tough Questions.* June 30, 2014.

49 Carl Brenner, *Explanation of the Lyme Disease Western Blot,* December 13, 1999. http://www.lymenet.de/labtests/brenner.htm

50 Lesley Fein, Shawn Bean, Jess Armine Blog Talk Radio Show, *Lyme Disease: Open Mic Night: Time to ask the Tough Questions.* June 30, 2014.

51 Jess Armine, Blog Talk Radio Show, *Lyme Disease: the 411!* June 23, 2014.

52 Lesley Fein, Shawn Bean, Jess Armine Blog Talk Radio Show, *Lyme Disease: Open Mic Night: Time to ask the Tough Questions.* June 30, 2014.

53 Ibid

54 http://canlyme.com/for-physicians/

55 http://www.guideline.gov/content.aspx? id=49320

56 http://canlyme.com/wp-content/uploads/guidelines/BurrGuide200810.pdf

Chapter 2

57 Jess Armine, Blog Talk Radio Show, *POTS...the 411!* February 2, 2015 http://methylationsupport.com/dev/podcasts/

58 Panache Desai, *21-Day Ultimate Energy Immersion Program*, group phone call, Sept. 10, 2015.

59 Peggy Kornegger, *21-Day Ultimate Energy Immersion Program*, group phone call, Sept. 10, 2015.

Chapter 3

60 Austin Kleon, *Steal Like an Artist*, in Brian Johnson's Philosopher's Notes.

61 https://en.wikipedia.org/wiki/E-patient

62 http://www.ted.com/talks/dave_debronkart_meet_e_patient_dave?language=en#t-954306

63 http://e-patients.net/archives/2015/10/when-someone-else-speaks-for-you-you-lose-patient-empowerment-as-a-civil-rights-movement.html

64 Jess Armine, Blog Talk Radio Show, *POTS...the 411!* February 2, 2015. http://methylationsupport.com/dev/podcasts/

65 Medical Intuition: Lori Wilson's Total Body Intuition™ Foundation Level http://www.inneraccess101.com/Copy%20of%20medical_foundation.htm

66 Lori Wilson: *demystifying...Medical Intuition.* (Toronto: Lori Wilson, 2005).

67 Shawn Bean, Matrix Health and Wellness LLC, http://matrixhealthwell.com/, personal communication, October 2014.

Chapter 4

68 http://www.brainyquote.com/quotes/quotes/c/christophe141891.html?src=t_overwhelming

69 http://criticalhealthfacts.com/dying-of-lyme-disease-case-fatality-rate-nearly-100/

70 Tynan, Superhuman by Habit https://brianjohnson. me/philosophersnotes/the-books/?wpv_paged_ preload_reach=1&wpv_view_count=47634-40cd750b- ba9870f18aada2478b24840a&wpv_post_ id=133&pn-author-name%5B0%5D=Tynan&wpv_ filter_submit=Search&wpv_post_search

71 Gabor Maté, *When the Body Says No.* (Toronto: Vintage Canada, 2003).

72 Peter Levine, *In an Unspoken Voice: How the Body Releases Trauma and Restores Goodness.* (Berkeley: North Atlantic Books, 2010).

73 V Felitti et al, *Relationship of Childhood Abuse and Household Dysfunction to Many of the Leading Causes of Death in Adults: The Adverse Childhood Experiences (ACE) Study.* Amer. J Prev. Med., Vol 14, Issue 4, Pages 245–258, May 1998. http://www.ajpmonline. org/article/S0749-3797(98)00017-8/fulltext

74 Irene Lyon, *Why Mindfulness Practices Don't Work— Learning the Groundwork to Meditation.* https:// irenelyon.com/2014/04/18/mindfulness-practic- es-dont-always-work-learning-groundwork-medita- tion/.

Chapter 5

75 Jill Bolte Taylor, interview with Oprah Winfrey, *Super Soul Sunday* TV program July 26, 2015.

76 Fawne Hansen, *How Does Stress affect your Immune System?* July 20, 2014. http://adrenalfatiguesolution. com/stress-immune-system/

77 Marcelle Pick, *Are You Tired And Wired?* (New York: Hay House, 2011).

78 Amy Myers, *The Autoimmune Solution.* (New York: HarperCollins, 2015).

79 Annie Hopper, *Wired For Healing.* (Victoria: The Dynamic Neural Retraining System™, 2014).

80 Stephen W. Porges, *The Polyvagal Theory: Neurophysiological Foundations of Emotions, Attachment, Communication, and Self-regulation (Norton Series on Interpersonal Neurobiology)* (New York: W. W. Norton & Company, 2011).

81 Irene Lyon, *An Epidemic of Chronic Illness: How Stress, Trauma & Adversity Early in Life Impacts Our Capacity to Heal.* https://irenelyon.com/2017/02/03/epidemic-chronic-illness-stress-trauma-adversity-early-life-impacts-capacity-heal/

82 Mark Wolynn: *It Didn't Start With You: How Inherited Family Trauma Shapes Who We Are And How To End The Cycle.* (New York: Viking, 2016).

83 Joe Dispenza, *Breaking the Habit of Being Yourself.* (New York: Hay House, 2012).

84 Norman Doidge, *The Brain's Way of Healing: Remarkable Discoveries and Recoveries from the Frontiers of Neuroplasticity.* (New York: Viking, 2015)

85 Bessel Van der Kolk: *The Body Keeps the Score: Brain, Mind and Body in the Healing of Trauma.* (New York: Viking, 2014)

86 Gabor Maté, *When the Body Says No.* (Toronto: Vintage Canada, 2003).

87 Irene Lyon, *An Epidemic of Chronic Illness: How Stress, Trauma & Adversity Early in Life Impacts Our Capacity to Heal.* https://irenelyon.com/2017/02/03/epidemic-chronic-illness-stress-trauma-adversity-early-life-impacts-capacity-heal/

88 http://www.emofree.com/index.php?q=chronic+illness&option=com_finder&view=search&lang=en-US&Itemid=300

89 Peter Levine, *In an Unspoken Voice: How the Body Releases Trauma and Restores Goodness.* (Berkeley: North Atlantic Books, 2010), 48.

90 Joe Dispenza, *You Are the Placebo: Making Your Mind Matter.* (Carlsbad: Hay House, 2014)

Conclusion

91 http://www.oprah.com/own-own/In-Deep-Shift-with-Jonas-Elrod-Series-Premiere-February-8-Video

92 http://www.oprah.com/own-indeepshift/Jonas-Elrod-on-Breakdowns-and-Obstacles-Video)

Resources

Alan Christianson, The Adrenal Reset Diet, Strategically Cycle Carbs and Proteins to Lose Weight, Balance Hormones, and Move from Stressed to Thriving (New York: Harmony, 2014)

Julie Daniluk, *Hot Detox: A 21-Day Anti-Inflammatory Program to Heal Your Gut and Cleanse Your Body.* (Toronto: Harper Collins, 2016).

William Davis, *Wheat Belly 30 Minute (or Less!) Cookbook*, (Toronto: Harper Collins, 2013).

Amy Myers, *The Autoimmune Solution*, (New York: HarperCollins, 2015).

JJ Virgin, *The Virgin Diet*, (Don Mills: Harlequin, 2012).

Terry Wahls, *The Wahls Protocol*, (New York: Penguin, 2014).

David Perlmutter, *Brain Maker*, (New York: Little, Brown and Company, 2015).

Paul Frewen, Ph. D., Ruth Lanius, Ph. D. *Healing the Traumatized Self: Consciousness, Neuroscience, Treatment* (Norton Series on Interpersonal Neurobiology) (New York: W. W. Norton & Company, 2015).

Rick Hanson, *Hardwiring Happiness: The New Brain Science*

of Contentment, Calm, and Confidence (New York: Random House, 2013).

Peter A. Levine, Ph. D., *In an Unspoken Voice: How the Body Releases Trauma and Restores Goodness* (Berkeley: North Atlantic Books, 2012).

Stephen W. Porges, *The Polyvagal Theory: Neurophysiological Foundations of Emotions, Attachment, Communication, and Self-regulation* (Norton Series on Interpersonal Neurobiology) (New York: W. W. Norton & Company, 2011).

Bessel Van der Kolk: *The Body Keeps the Score: Brain, Mind and Body in the Healing of Trauma.* (New York: Viking, 2014)

Gabor Maté, *When the Body Says No.* (Toronto: Vintage Canada, 2003).

Irene Lyon, *Dr. Peter Levine, the Founder of Somatic Experiencing explains how the human system can heal and self-regulate from traumatic events.* https://irenelyon. com/2010/12/22/titrate-this-dr-peter-levine-the-founder-of-somatic-experiencing-explains-how-the-human-system-can-heal-and-self-regulate-from-traumatic-events/

Richard I. Horowitz, *How Can I Get Better? An Action Plan for Treating Resistant Lyme & Chronic Disease.* (New York: St. Martin's Griffin, 2017)

Katina Makriss, *Autoimmune Illness and Lyme Disease Recovery Guide: Mending the Body, Mind and Spirit.* (New York: Helios Press, 2015).

Acknowledgments

I would like to thank all of my patients and clients over the past 40+ years who have entrusted me to be a guide and co-pilot in your precious care and well-being. You have constantly inspired me with your innate wisdom and well-earned experience, and fueled my awe and wonder about all that creates health and illness.

Thank you to Joan Ross, Lori Wilson, Lynda Buckland and Rebecca Liston, for your loving presence in my life. It means the world to me.

Anne Marie Heron, thank you for so many years of loving friendship and for making your pivotal statement not long ago, "You should write a book. Really!"

Thank you to Panache Desai, Sue Simcox and my other online and non-physical family members of vibrationally present beings. My light is shining stronger with your support.

To my many skilled health care professionals past and present, thank you for doing your best and for the valuable part each of you have played in my health care journey and personal learning. A special thanks to Shawn Bean, Dr. Jess Armine and Dr. Lesley Fein for opening the door to a level of health care expertise and fierce determination that

I thought existed only in my imagination.

Cindy Shrigley, Gary Blier, Doris Vargas, and Irene Lyon, you are rocking the world with your talent and contribution in your respective fields. You have changed my life with your innovative approaches to healing.

To Kevin Nations and Melissa Nations, my heartfelt thanks for holding your strong beliefs in vision, excellence and action. Your timely personal support in some of my key life decisions has meant far more than you know.

Kate Makled, thank you for holding that important space of faith, expression and completion, along with your skills of editorial elevation. We did it!

Angela Lauria, my initial publisher and inspiring book coach, thank you for your enthusiastic support and for living the expression of your personal mission. If you had not courageously acted upon what you have been called to do in your life, this book would not exist.

Thanks to my amazing Author Incubator cohort of authors past, present and future for your part in holding the collective vision of our deep self-expression and impactful serving of our respective readers and clients.

Thanks, from the bottom of my heart, to my husband Jeff Clendenning, for your unwavering support, faith and love that you have constantly demonstrated to me in every way possible for 29 years. You are a treasure beyond words.

About the Author

Lisa Dennys is an author, life coach and intuitive practitioner who has worked in health care and personal transformation fields since 1977. Her previous professional careers as a Dr. of Chinese Medicine & Acupuncture and an Occupational Therapist have given her a unique, holistic perspective on health and illness.

For over 30 years Lisa has dealt with her own serious health concerns, resulting in significant and devastating symptoms that at times completely disrupted all aspects of her life and work. A determined health detective, Lisa sought answers within and outside of the conventional medical system. After several decades of exhaustive and frustrating self-directed investigation and misdiagnosis, she was finally diagnosed with chronic Lyme disease in early 2015. Her long path to a diagnosis and now finally into treatment and recovery has encompassed many challenging experiences and created deep personal transformation.

An insatiable life-long reader and student of life, personal growth and health, Lisa applies her unique, comprehensive tools and broad perspective to help her clients ask probing questions and seek deeper answers. She supports and guides people with complex chronic illness, including those with chronic Lyme disease, to build a skilled professional treatment team, navigate the medical system and look inward for intuitive answers — *to find out for sure what is really going on* — and to finally answer the question, *Is This What's Behind Your Chronic Illness?*

Lisa and her beloved husband Jeff Clendenning live with their dog and cat family in Sarnia, Ontario, Canada.

Thank You
Complimentary Resources for Readers

Dear Reader,

Thanks so much for reading my book! I wish you the very best as you go further on your journey towards finding answers for your challenging health situation.

As a thank you and to help you take the next step in applying the information in this book, I've prepared some bonus materials for you.

Your Quick Start Guide to Unveiling Lyme Disease can be accessed here www.unveilinglyme.com/thankyou and consists of:

- **A self-questionnaire,** formulated by Lyme specialist Richard I. Horowitz MD, author of *Why Can't I Get Better? Solving the Mystery of Lyme & Chronic Disease*, to help you and your health care professional determine if your unique symptoms may possibly fit the pattern of Lyme disease

- **Self-screening checklists** to help you determine if you're ready to take the next steps to pursuing a new medical diagnosis on your own, or whether you need further support

- **Three audios of my 1 on 1 client coaching sessions** dealing with the challenges of pursuing a diagnosis of Lyme

- **An audio of my Tele-seminar,** *"Could Lyme Disease be the Cause of Your Chronic Illness?"*

- **Resource list** of practitioners, links, and further reading

Here's that link again to access your complimentary materials: www.unveilinglyme.com/thankyou

Looking for 1 on 1 help…now?

If you'd like some expertise and guidance on your determined path to better health, and you want to get there as quickly and efficiently as possible, I can help. This link will take you directly to detailed information about how you can get support from me as your coach:

www.unveilinglyme.com/workwithlisa.

You can also email me at info@unveilinglyme.com.